Acknowledgements

Extensive use has been made of the publications of a number of authors who are well known for their interest in spina bifida, and although these are referred to in the text and listed at the end of the book, my indebtedness extends beyond this and I would like to express here my acknowlegement of these authorities.

A number of important contributions to the subject of spina bifida have been generated by the meetings of the Society for Research into Hydrocephalus and Spina Bifida. The proceedings of these meetings have been published as supplements to *Developmental Medicine and Child Neurology* since 1965 by Spastics International Medical Publications. The important rôle of these organisations and the helpful co-operation of Dr. Martin Bax is acknowledged.

Finally, I would like to acknowledge the diligent help of my secretaries — Ann Milton and Susan Smith — in the preparation and typing of this book.

AUTHORS' APPOINTMENTS

Gordon Brocklehurst

Consultant Neurosurgeon,
Hull Royal Infirmary,
Hull HU3 2JZ

Duncan Forrest

Consultant Paediatric Surgeon,
Westminster Children's Hospital,
Vincent Square,
London SW1

Queen Mary's Hospital for Sick Children,
Carshalton,
Surrey

Children's Hospital,
Sydenham Road,
Sydenham,
London SE26 5ER

W. J. W. Sharrard

Consultant Orthopaedic Surgeon,
Sheffield Children's Hospital,
King Edward VII Hospital, Rivelin
and Sheffield Royal Infirmary

Gordon Stark

Consultant Paediatrician,
Royal Hospital for Sick Children,
Department of Child Life and Health,
Edinburgh EH9 1UW

SPINA BIFIDA FOR THE CLINICIAN

Clinics in Developmental Medicine No. 57

Spina Bifida for the Clinician

Edited by

GORDON BROCKLEHURST

1976

Spastics International Medical Publications

LONDON: William Heinemann Medical Books Ltd.

PHILADELPHIA: J. B. Lippincott Co.

LR L J (M)

ISBN 0 433 04410 1

Printed in England at THE LAVENHAM PRESS LTD., Lavenham, Suffolk

BROCKLEHURST

copy 2

Introduction

During the last 20 years the condition of spina bifida has been subjected to one of those swings of the pendulum of interest which so frequently occur in medicine. The disappearance of tuberculosis and poliomyelitis as major problems in childhood has permitted more attention to be paid to congenital malformations, and recent advances in surgical technique and management have made treatment of the open spina bifida lesion and the associated hydrocephalus a practical possibility.

The initial enthusiasm demonstrated in the 1950s and 1960s for the surgical treatment of infants with spina bifida lesions has now been tempered by the recognition that among the survivors are many who carry combined mental and physical disabilities of great severity into later childhood. The value of the therapeutic industry which led to the prolongation of such limited lives is now seriously questioned.

On the other hand, the renewed interest in the condition has stimulated a more detailed examination of the pathology and clinical features; the wide variety of lesions of the central nervous system and other structures found in association with spina bifida is now well recognised, and the necessity for a full examination and assessment of the individual patient presenting with the condition is acknowledged. Furthermore, the experience accumulated during the last 20 years of comprehensive and detailed treatment of spina bifida patients can now be included in considering the prognosis for any particular infant.

The recent efforts to provide concerned parents with more relevant genetic counselling in this and other conditions, and the attempts to diagnose the condition *in utero* sufficiently early to consider therapeutic abortion are both steps towards the ultimate goal of prevention. Until this goal is achieved many infants will continue to be born with a variety of spina bifida lesions; each child will merit accurate appreciation of the accompanying neurological disability, and clear advice should be offered to the parents regarding prognosis and treatment. When treatment is undertaken, a team consisting of the paediatrician, neurosurgeon, orthopaedic and urological surgeons, family practitioner, nursing staff, physiotherapist, social worker and parents will be involved; the repercussions of the undertaking will be borne by the family and the local community. Special hospital and educational facilities will be required, and some administrative arrangements made to finance this kind of comprehensive care.

This book aims to provide an understanding of the nature, pathology, clinical presentation, and clinical management of spina bifida sufficient to aid practitioners with their assessment and care of these patients, and in reaching a reasonably accurate prognosis so that appropriate advice can be given to the parents of such a child.

Gordon Brocklehurst

Contents

CHAPTER 1

The Nature of Spina Bifida

Tulp and Morgagni

Nicholas Tulp, the teacher portrayed in Rembrandt's 'The Anatomy Lesson', 1632, was the author of the first concise description of spina bifida. Figure 1.1 is taken from the 1652 edition of his book entitled 'Observationes Medicae'. Tulp clearly recognised the involvement of the central nervous system in the swelling on the infant's back ('nervorum propagines tam varie per tumorem dispersas') and he also appreciated the dire consequences of incising such a 'tumor'.

The term 'spina bifida' which Tulp applied to this condition has remained a useful one, since it describes the feature common to a large group of malformations, namely, the separation of the vertebral elements in the midline.

It was Morgagni in 1761 who first clearly linked hydrocephalus with spina bifida under the heading 'Sermo de Hydrocephalus et de Aqueis Spinae Tumoribus' in his classical book 'De sedibus et Causis Morborum per Anatomen Indigatis'. He described many types of acute and chronic forms of hydrocephalus and linked these with the fluid-filled spina bifida tumour; he also noted that either condition might occur singly. The anatomy and physiology of the cerebrospinal fluid was not appreciated at the time when Morgagni was writing and his phrase 'hydrops cerebri et medullaris' can only be interpreted literally, or, as William Cooke translated it in 1822, 'there is naturally a little fluid in the spinal canal and should this exceed the natural quantity it may be considered as an occasion of hydro-rachitis'. The attribution to Morgagni of the concept that spina bifida is actually caused by hydrocephalus is an overstatement somewhat determined by later views of the pathology of the cerebrospinal fluid. On the other hand, the very close association between hydrocephalus and nearly all forms of spina bifida has been amply confirmed, and the aetiological relationship of the one to the other will be discussed in later chapters.

William Cooke, in the editorial comments on his translation of Morgagni's *magnum opus,* described a patient with spina bifida 'killed by the knife' and quoted Sir Astley Cooper as stating that the treatment of spina bifida was either 'palliative, by pressure, or curative, by puncture'. This dynamic relationship between the incentive of possible methods of treatment and the endeavour to understand the pathogenisis is a recurrent feature in any historical survey of the literature upon spina bifida (Brocklehurst 1971).

The Nineteenth Century

Lamarck's account of the effect of environment upon development and heredity was published in 1809, and by 1836 Geoffroy St. Hilaire had completed his compilation and classification of monstrosities in which he related these to each other

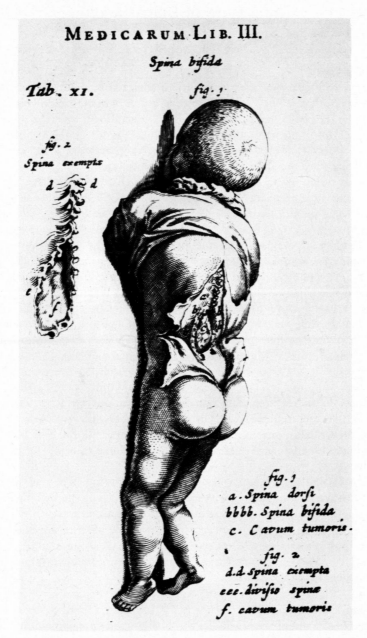

Figure 1.1. Spina bifida. Illustration taken from 'Observationes Medicae' by Nicholas Tulp, Amsterdam 1652.

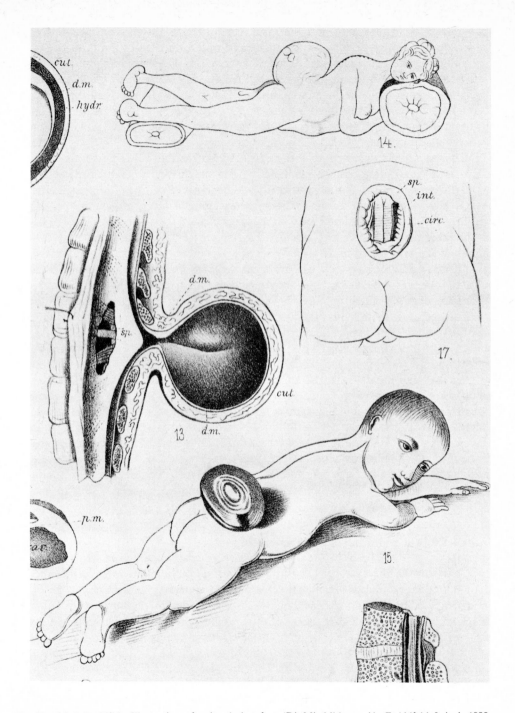

Fig. 1.2. Spina bifida. Illustrations of various lesions from 'Die Missbildungen' by F. Ahlfeld. Leipzig 1880.

as species within genera, thus promoting the concept that monsters were caused by a modification of the embryo by environment and were examples of the influence of environment on heredity. Darwin's account of the origin of species was published in 1859 and by this time the details of the embryology of the nervous system and its development from the neural tube were also well established. By the 1860s onwards, therefore, the occurrence of malformations of the nervous system could be related to the normal stages of development and interpreted with either a Darwinian or Lamarckian approach.

Virchow (1863) observed that the cystic lesion on the back of the common lumbar and sacral spina bifida cases had a central pit; this, he thought, marked the unusually low end of the spinal cord which had been prevented from undergoing its normal relative retraction during embryonic development by its attachment to the wall of the cyst. He considered that the basic pathogenesis was an excess of fluid within the central canal of the spinal cord, termed 'hydromyelia', and that this caused, in the majority of spina bifida cases, a cystic dilatation at the tail end of the spinal cord, with a consequent herniation through the vertebrae and tissues of the back. In other cases the hydromyelia became obstructed by adhesions situated more proximally and the dilatation then caused a cervical or occipital 'myelocele' or 'encephalocele.' Ahlfeld, in his massive compilation of malformations, tabulated and illustrated in 1880 (see Fig. 1.2), also took the view that an excess of fluid caused the majority of spina bifida cases ('Man muss für die Mehrzahl der Fälle die primäre Ursache im spinalen Hydrops suchen').

On the other hand, Lebedeff, at a similar time (1881, 1882), emphasised that spina bifida was caused by a failure of the neural tube to close during early embryological development ('Entstehung der Hemicephalie und Spina Bifida zurück auf Anomalie Krümmungen des Medullarrohrs in der frühesten fötalen Periode') and was accompanied by an overgrowth of the medullary blastema. Thus, by the last two decades of the nineteenth century there were added to the 'hydrops cerebri et medullaris' concept of Morgagni those of 'failure-to-fuse', 'neural overgrowth' and 'spinal cord tethering' in the endeavours to approach an understanding of the pathogenesis of spina bifida.

Morton, Cleland and The London Committee

Meanwhile, in Britain, Morton had begun to practise a method of treatment of spina bifida by the injection into the 'tumour' of a solution of iodine in glycerine, and in 1877 the first edition of his book on this method appeared. Individual reports of patients treated by the iodo-glycerine injection were quite frequent between 1870 and 1880 and it seems probable that this spate of so-called 'surgical' treatment stimulated interest in spina bifida again. Certainly, in 1883, there appeared a 'Contribution to the Study of Spina Bifida, Encephalocoele, and Anencephalus' by John Cleland, who mentioned the work of Dr. Morton in Glasgow, and, furthermore, contributed a whole chapter on the pathology of spina bifida to the 1887 edition of Morton's book.

Cleland's 1883 paper was a masterpiece of anatomical description combined with deductions which were clearly influenced by the work of St. Hilaire, Lebedeff and Ahlfeld, among others. The spina bifida specimen was that of a full-term infant with

4

a lesion which extended from the sixth thoracic to the first sacral vertebra. Cleland noted that the laminae of the second and third sacral vertebrae below the lesion were normally aligned, that the left third and fourth ribs were fused together, and that the membraneous bones of the skull contained circular perforations (craniolacunae). The skin over the spina bifida was deficient and the centre of this region occupied by a 'membraneous area', from the ventral side of which the nerve roots ran to their respective foramina. The membraneous area (neural plaque) had subarachnoid space around its ventral and lateral sides and a small aperture at its upper end. The spinal cord above the neural plaque contained a dilated central canal, the upper end of which terminated ¼ inch below the fourth ventricle. The fourth ventricle itself was clearly described as extending downwards into the cervical spinal canal for a distance of 1½ inches, and the caudal end of the fourth ventricle terminated in an imperforate depression.

The cerebellum in the posterior cranial fossa was deformed superiorly, so that the pyramid touched the corpora quadrigemina and the uvula faced backwards; inferiorly, the 'velum posticum' was caudally prolonged and the 'laminated tubercle' (nodule) hung down from this into the cavity of the fourth ventricle. In addition to this classical account of the brainstem deformity (which later became known as the 'Arnold-Chiari malformation'), Cleland described a deformity of the corpora quadrigemina with 'the testes projected above the nates, and the nates flattened' (a deformity which has since become known as 'tectal beaking'). These observations by Cleland thus include the salient malformations of neurectodermal and mesodermal origin associated with a typical open spina bifida lesion and included in such terms as 'spina bifida aperta' or 'cystica', 'myeloschisis', 'myelomeningocele', 'myelocele' and 'rachischisis' (see Chapter 3).

The observations upon the other conditions included in Cleland's study add further features of cerebral maldevelopment, including the completely open ventricular system of anencephalus, encephaloceles involving the fourth ventricle and cerebellum, other vertebral malformations such as anterior spina bifida and hemivertebrae, the occurrence of nodules of cerebral tumour accompanying the spinal malformations (heteroplasia), and the absence of viscera in some of the most severe examples. Moving from observation to hypothesis, Cleland followed the thought of St. Hilaire and linked all of these monstrosities together under the common factor of 'the modification of the embryo by environment'. Considering the pathogenesis in more detail, Cleland postulated that some change in the environment of the early embryo caused an undue stimulation of growth, and that this led either to an excessive production of fluid within the embryo and consequent rupture of the neural tube to produce anencephalus, encephalocele, hydrocephalus or myelomeningocele (depending upon the actual time of the rupture), or to a disproportionate growth of the nervous tissue compared with the surrounding mesoderm, producing buckling of the tube and failure to fuse.

Cleland's concepts were thus not only a superb integration of anatomy, pathology, and embryology of the 1880s, but were also compatible with the contemporary understanding of teratology and biology. Many subsequent observations and hypotheses concerned with spina bifida have approached the subject from a more limited aspect and it is now beset with a bewildering array of conflicting views (Brocklehurst 1971).

Further evidence of the nineteenth century interest in spina bifida that was engendered by the Morton method of treatment was the appointment in 1882, by the Clinical Society of London, of a distinguished committee to investigate spina bifida and its treatment by the injection of Dr. Morton's iodo-glycerine solution. The Committee reported in 1885 and provided valuable information on the clinical features of 236 cases of spina bifida and pathological findings in 125 specimens from various museums throughout the country; they showed a full appreciation of the pathology and considered that in 70 per cent of the 'tumours' the spinal cord or nerve roots were in the sac, and that the split spinal cord was the basis of the malformation of the nervous system. With regard to treatment, the London Committee made valuable observations upon the death rate from spina bifida (indicating that about one per cent survive without treatment), and also upon the state of 60 untreated patients, and the results of various methods of treatment, among which Morton's method had proved to be the most satisfactory (Marsh *et al.* 1885).

In the same volume of the London Clinical Society's transactions there appeared a paper by Mayo Robson (1885), reporting a method of surgical excision and plastic closure of the spina bifida lesion with some successful results, but the London Committee was opposed to this because of the nerve roots contained in the sac of the tumour.

Professor Humphry in Cambridge shared in the current interest in spina bifida and in 1885 produced a beautifully-worded description of the appearances of spina bifida lesions. He explained accurately the relationship of the nerves and neural plaque to the meningocele sac, and noted the transverse course of the nerves from the middle of the plaque to their foramina and the cephalic direction of the uppermost nerves. In the same year, Humphry's lecture entitled 'Six specimens of spina bifida with bony projections from the bodies of the vertebral canal' was published: this contained a fine description of the bony spurs which accompany the partial duplication of the spinal cord. (This partial duplication sometimes occurs in conjunction with spina bifida and is called 'diastematomyelia'—see Chapter 3.) Humphry's views on the pathogenesis of these conditions oscillated between the hydrops medullaris and failure-to-fuse concepts, and his accurate descriptions of the bony spurs and hemi-vertebrae remain a classical record.

Thus, by 1890, there existed in Great Britain authoritative observations and views upon many aspects of spina bifida, and in the stimulation of these views the possibility of some form of treatment of the condition appears to have played no small part. However, when Dr. Morton's reports are read carefully, it is clear that the initial results of the treatment, even if acceptable, are far outweighed by the very considerable problems of hydrocephalus, infection, incontinence and paraplegia, and it is not surprising that enthusiasm for this treatment did not persist.

The Occult Forms of Spina Bifida
While surgical enthusiasm waned the contributions to the study of spina bifida

from the increasingly scientific disciplines of pathology, embryology and teratology, began to accumulate.

In 1886, von Recklinghausen described an adult with a spina bifida lesion that was covered by skin and an excess of hair (spina bifida occulta and lumbosacral hypertrichosis). The patient had suffered from a club foot with an anaesthetic ulcer which led to osteomyelitis, amputation, septicaemia and death. The post-mortem examination showed that the spinal canal was widened from the fifth lumbar vertebra downwards and contained a fatty tumour in the lumbo-sacral region over which was stretched the conus medullaris (which ended at the second sacral vertebra) and the sacral nerve roots. He related the clinical manifestations of spina bifida occulta (hypertrichosis over the sacral region and the club foot) to the descriptions of satyrs with tails and hooves so common in mythology, and the pathological findings of the lesion he related to those which occur in the open spina bifida cases. He considered that the case which he studied was an example of a disturbance of neural tube closure in which the lipoma arose from some abnormality in the separation of mesodermal elements during embryological development, and the previously open myelomeningocele became closed during later fetal development.

In discussing the spinal cord lesions which accompany spina bifida in general, he differed from the London Committee, and rather than accept the split spinal cord (rachischisis or myeloschisis) as the basic feature, he concluded that the neural tube closed and the cord became part of the sac wall of the cystic swelling ('Tumor der Spina Bifida seine Höhle innerhalb der Arachnoidea bildet'). Von Recklinghausen's view is important in drawing attention to the variety of lesion associated with spina bifida occulta which is compatible with a long post-natal survival without treatment, and can be entirely dissociated from hydrocephalus. His interpretation of the spina bifida 'tumor' in the open lesions as an accumulation of fluid within the subarachnoid space is also important (see Chapter 3).

Arnold, Chiari and the Brainstem Malformation

The historical origin of the eponym for the brainstem malformation now classically associated with spina bifida requires some appreciation in order that the term may be used with appropriate accuracy. Chiari's contribution is the most complex: in 1891 he published from Prague a series of initial observations upon what he called 'deformity of the cerebellum as a result of hydrocephalus' ('Über Veranderungen des Kleinhirns infolge von Hydrocephalie des Grosshirns'), and gave examples of what he considered to be three different types. In 1896 he published a well-illustrated monograph in which he enlarged upon his concepts and included more examples of the types.

Type I, of which 14 examples were given, was characterised by prolongation of the cerebellar *tonsils* and the most medial part of the inferior lobe of the cerebellum (Fig. 1.3). All 14 patients had ventricular dilatation, and most had possible causes of hydrocephalus such as tuberculous, carcinomatous or pyogenic meningitis. There was only one case of spina bifida in this group, a child aged two years, and the description of the hindbrain clearly conforms to Type I, although the findings were not included in the illustrations.

7

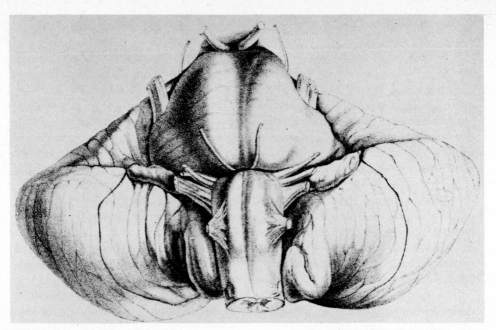

Fig. 1.3. Chiari's Type I brainstem malformation (chronic tonsillar herniation). Illustration from Wien Denkschrift Akademische Wissenschaft, 1896.

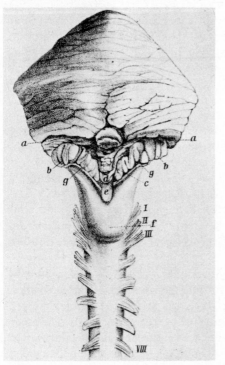

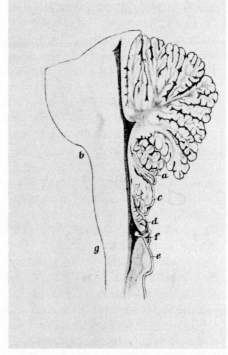

Fig. 1.4. Chiari's Type 2 brainstem malformation (congenital malformation of cerebellar vermis associated with spina bifida). Illustration from Wien Denkschrift Akademische Wissenschaft, 1896.

In Chiari's Type II deformity, the prolongation involved the cerebellar *vermis*, not the tonsils, and was associated with inferior prolongation of the fourth ventricle into the cervical spinal canal and with kinking of the inferiorly displaced medulla oblongata (Fig. 1.4). Seven examples of this type of deformity were presented and all had extensive spina bifida.

In Type III the deformity was more extensive and the dilated fourth ventricle and cerebellum were found within the sac of a cervical encephalocele: the one example of this type was the same as that described in the 1891 communication. A Type IV was added in the 1896 monograph and in this the outstanding feature was cerebellar hypoplasia: one example had an encephalocele and none had spina bifida.

Chiari noted Cleland's observations and concluded that all of the cerebellar malformations were due to hydrocephalus. Subsequent knowledge of cerebrospinal fluid physiology and pathology suggest that Chiari's view was correct in the case of Type I: this is a description of chronic tonsillar herniation which is known to follow many varieties of raised intracranial pressure, including chronic hydrocephalus. Type II is a much more extensive malformation involving the cerebellar vermis and other brainstem structures, and it still remains to be demonstrated that pressure differentials can develop *in utero* at a sufficiently early stage in the embryology of the hindbrain to produce such an extensive plastic deformity. The alternative explanation is that Types II, III and IV are primary brainstem malformations and are aetiologically independent of hydrocephalus. The high degree of association of the Type II deformity with spina bifida has been amply confirmed, and the occurrence of less severe brainstem malformations as primary deformities without spina bifida has also been frequently described.

In 1894, Arnold described the pathological findings in an infant who died shortly after birth and displayed a gross spina bifida 'tumor' in the thoraco-lumbar region with associated sympodia and massive dysplasia of tissues of mesodermal origin. The spinal bifida extended from the ninth thoracic vertebra downwards, and the bodies of the seventh and eighth thoracic vertebrae were also abnormal. He interpreted the 'tumor' as a 'myelocyst', with strands of cord tissue going into the sac, and he identified smaller tumours of mesodermal origin in the fundus and neck of the sac. He noted that the brainstem was poorly developed and that there was prolongation of the cerebellum over the roof of the fourth ventricle, completely covering this structure, and this deformed brainstem was situated in the cervical spinal canal ('Kleinhirn nach unten in eine bandartige Masse fort, welche oben breiter, unten schmäler ist und den IV ventricle vollständig bedeckend beinahe bis zur Mitte des Cervicalmarks herabreicht'). He specifically noted that the ventricles of the cerebral hemispheres were not enlarged (Fig. 1.5).

In a lengthy discussion, Arnold quoted the views of von Recklinghausen and noted the findings of the London Committee. He also considered Morgagni's concept of hydrops cerebri et medullaris, but finally concluded that his own observations indicated a primary disturbance in the organisation of germ layers resulting in a 'monogerminal teratomatous malformation': he made no particular extension of this concept to include the hindbrain malformation.

It was Schwalbe and Gredig, pupils of Arnold, who in 1907 re-emphasized the

9

close association of the hindbrain malformations with spina bifida, and coined the term 'Arnoldsche und Chiarische Missbildung'. The prime purpose of their contribution was to emphasize that the majority of cases of spina bifida showed this malformation to some degree, and in discussing the paucity of previous literature on the subject, their failure to notice Cleland's contribution is made more apparent. They described four infants with spina bifida (two thoraco-lumbar and two lumbo-sacral), all with hypoplasia of the cerebellum and pons, downward displacement and dorsal kinking of the medulla (the so-called 'Knickung') over the upper cervical spinal cord, and prolongation of hypoplastic cerebellar vermis into, or over, an elongated fourth ventricle. They noted also heterotopia of the cerebellum, associated with metaplasia, and that these latter features were sometimes found in cases without spina bifida. Enlargement, splitting and irregularity of the central canal was also described by these authors.

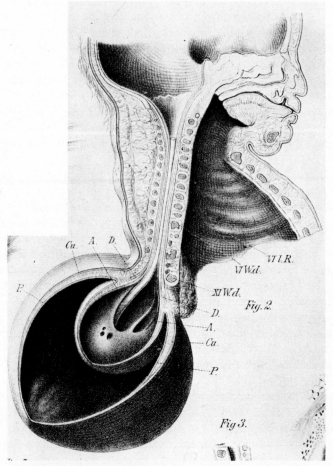

Fig. 1.5. Arnold's spina bifida case with sympodia and gross brainstem malformation. Illustration from 'Beitrage zur pathologischen Anatomie und zur allgemeinen Pathologie', 1894.

In their discussion on these hindbrain malformations Schwalbe and Gredig suggested a re-grouping into five degrees of severity: Group I was the most severe, and the prolongation of the vermis extended into the low fourth ventricle and the central canal; and Group V merely had an insignificant projection of cerebellar vermis caudally into the spinal canal. They took the view that spina bifida resulted from a very early disturbance in the development of the midline region of the nervous system at the site where the neural crests come together to form the neural tube; the brainstem malformation, they thought, was a disturbance of the development of the cerebellar anlage (Group I earliest and Group V latest), which occurred *after* the establishment of the spina bifida lesion and independently of it.

Developmental Pathology in the Early Twentieth Century

There is an important but small amount of early twentieth century literature upon the development of the neural tube which establishes the closure of the posterior neuropore by the 25-somite stage (*i.e.* when the embryo is 3.4mm in length) and this means that the lower lumbar and sacral spinal cord segments and accompanying mesodermal segments develop from the distal lip of the neuropore in relation to the tail-bud, and are not formed from the neural groove. These features have been related to the type of neural lesions which accompany spina bifida in the lumbo-sacral region (Holmdahl 1925). In 1929, Sternberg described a number of embryological specimens with abnormalities of closure in the neural tube and established some of the earliest stages at which these malformations become apparent. Grünewald, in 1941, described in detail a 20mm embryo with duplication of the spinal cord in the lower thoracic region accompanied by a thoraco-lumbar myeloschisis and a further antero-posterior duplication of the spinal cord in the sacral region. There were abnormalities of curvature of the vertebral column in this embryo and foci of dystopic tissue in the sacral region which contained nerve bundles, cartilage and nephroic tubules. He concluded that these abnormalities were of neural crest origin and he also noted that in this embryo there were no abnormal features in the head region. Ostertag, in reviewing the current concepts in 1956, related all of the midline malformations of the central nervous system to disturbances in the closure of the neural tube at different stages during the first four weeks of embryological development, thus maintaining the views of Lebedeff, von Recklinghausen and Arnold.

The Traction Theory

In 1938, Penfield and Coburn published a paper on the Arnold-Chiari malformation and its operative treatment. From the experience of a single patient who presented with evidence of brainstem compression (having had a thoraco-lumbar meningocele treated by operation some years earlier), they concluded that the Chiari Type II malformation, which they observed at a posterior fossa exploration, was due to traction. In the post-mortem examination of this case they noted that the cervical nerve roots ran in a cephalic direction and concluded that the spina bifida lesion had fixed the spinal cord during its development, and the normal relative upward movement of the conus medullaris was replaced by a downward movement of the brainstem. This was a further development of Virchow's concept. Lichtenstein, in

1940, described various examples of 'spinal dysraphism', all of which he considered were the result of failure of the neural tube to close normally, and in 1942 he described the 'distant neuro-anatomic complications' of spinal dysraphism such as aqueduct stenosis, brainstem malformation and hydrocephalus, all of which he considered to be due to tethering of the spinal cord. Ogryzlo (1942) and Ingraham and Scott (1943) took the same view, and it is clear that this hypothesis, which provides incentive for posterior fossa decompression, or for releasing the caudal tethering of the spinal cord, has continued to appeal to some surgeons (James and Lassman 1964, 1967).

A full dissection of a spina bifida specimen, illustrated in the paper by Ingraham and Scott (1943, *opus cit.*) shows that although the upper cervical nerves just caudal to the brainstem malformation do proceed in a cephalad direction, the lower cervical and thoracic nerve roots proceed in a relatively caudal direction to their exit foramina. At the level of the spina bifida lesion the roots proceed transversely or slightly cephalad. This macroscopic observation has been confirmed (Brocklehurst 1968a, 1969a, see Fig. 3.5), and measurements of the course of the nerve roots in spina bifida specimens have also demonstrated this feature (Barry *et al.* 1957; Brocklehurst 1968a, 1969a, *opera cit.*). If the spina bifida in these specimens had tethered the cord sufficiently to prevent its relative shortening, and thus pulled down the brainstem into the cervical spine, the intervening nerve roots would be expected to maintain their early embryological position in relation to their segmental vertebrae, and to proceed transversely to each of their respective foramina. The attenuation of the spinal cord immediately above the spina bifida lesion and the relatively normal course of the nerve roots in these upper segments suggest that this portion of the cord has indeed undergone relative shortening in normal fashion. Furthermore, in a recent experiment during which the lower end of the spinal cord in developing rats was fixed to the adjacent vertebrae, none of the few animals that survived the manipulation showed a brainstem malformation at full term (Goldstein and Kepes 1966).

The Overgrowth Hypothesis

In 1953, Patten described an 8mm human embryo with established myeloschisis and recorded that at the site of the myeloschisis the neural tube was everted and rather proud in appearance. He also reported a 49mm fetus with lumbo-sacral myeloschisis and a fully developed diastematomyelia caudal to the spina bifida, and a serially-sectioned, full-term rabbit fetus with myeloschisis. Using a squared microscope graticule, he compared the neural tissue in the latter specimen with that of a normal rabbit fetus and concluded that the lesion was due to overgrowth of the neural tissue, which is an extension of Lebedeff's concept.

In a later study concerned more with the associated brainstem malformation, Barry *et al.* (1957) studied the relationship between the neural tissue in three fetuses with myeloschisis and that in a normally developed neural tube. They observed that the volume of the neural tissue was greater at the level of the myeloschisis, but that the cord was relatively thinner on the cephalic side of the lesion. In the cervical region also, the abnormal fetuses had relatively more neural tissue. They added to these measurements the gross observation (without measurement) that the malformed medulla and cerebellum appeared large in relationship to the surrounding mesodermal structures comprising the skull, and they concluded that the malformation of the hindbrain and the associated deformities of the midbrain, and micropolygyria of the cerebral hemispheres were all caused by overgrowth of nervous tissue.

Encephalo-cranial Disproportion

This term was used by Doran and Guthkelch in 1961 to describe the apparent crowding of the neural tissue within the posterior fossa and upper cervical spine of patients with spina bifida, and it expresses the particular manifestation of the overgrowth hypothesis put forward by Patten (1953) and Barry *et al.* (1957).

In some recent observations (Brocklehurst 1968*a*, 1969*a*), measurements of a serially-sectioned spina bifida fetus of 95mm crown-rump length were made and compared with the same measurements in a 99mm normal fetus. The findings of Barry *et al.* (1957) with regard to the spinal cord were confirmed. However, when the contents of the posterior fossa in the two fetuses were actually measured, it was found that the posterior fossa of the abnormal fetus was very much smaller than that of the normal, and had deformed cerebellum and medulla crowded into it at the expense of the subarachnoid spaces (Fig. 1.6). Nevertheless, when the total volume of neural tissue from the pineal body to a similar level in the cervical spine of both fetuses was measured, the amount in the spina bifida fetus was less than half of that in the normal. It was concluded that the malformation was not one of overgrowth of neural tissue but of abnormal proportions between neurectoderm and surrounding mesoderm.

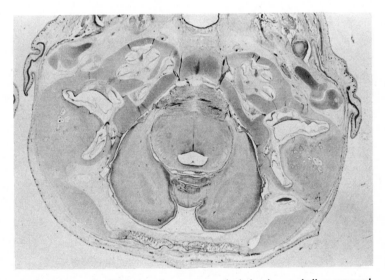

Fig. 1.6. 95mm spina bifida fetus (transverse section) showing cerebellum wrapped round upper part of fourth ventricle and deformed pons and brachium pontis. There is an apparent crowding of the hindbrain into the small posterior fossa. (From Brocklehurst 1969*a*.)

13

Teratology

Experimental teratologists have produced spina bifida and other malformations of the central nervous system by a variety of techniques. Fowler (1953) produced spina bifida in the chick by mechanical interference with the neural tube just after closure, and found that the myeloschisis was accompanied by apparent overgrowth of neural tissue. Warkany *et al.* (1958), using Trypan blue injections in pregnant rats, were able to produce various degrees of myeloschisis in the offspring, depending upon the actual time of gestation at which the teratogenic agent was administered: overgrowth and mesenchymal disorganisation were produced first, and a full myeloschisis with eversion of the neural tube later. These caudal deformities were accompanied by flattening of the fourth ventricle and caudal displacement of the cerebellum, so that the vermis protruded through the foramen magnum. Hydrocephalus was not evident in these offspring (Fig. 1.7).

Similar experiments using high Vitamin A diets in rats, birds and frogs (Giroud *et al.* 1960, 1961) produced anencephaly, encephalocele and myeloschisis accompanied by spina bifida. From a detailed study of the various stages in the malformation, they concluded that there was a disturbance in 'tissue organisers' which accompanied the non-closure of the neural tube, and this produced a failure of mesodermal fusion and disorganisation of the derivatives of both germ layers.

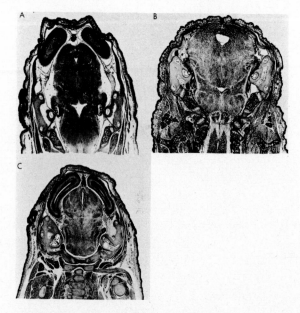

Fig. 1.7. Frontal sections through midbrain and hindbrain of rat fetuses (21st day). A—control, B and C—Trypan blue treated animals with spina bifida. B—marked crowding of cerebral tissue in skull. Note absence of cisternae. C—although there is crowding in the region of the midbrain and hindbrain, there is no hydrocephalus. (From Warkany 1971.)

14

CHAPTER 2

The Nature of the Hydrocephalus Associated with Spina Bifida

Classical Concepts of Cerebrospinal Fluid and Hydrocephalus

Knowledge of the anatomy, physiology and pathology of the cerebrospinal fluid (CSF) accumulated slowly during the nineteenth century, underwent a renaissance in the early twentieth century, and only now is its truly complex nature beginning to be appreciated. Cotugno, in 1769, observed that there was fluid around the brain and spinal cord as well as in the ventricular system, and Magendie, in a series of publications between 1825 and 1842, defined the communication of the ventricular and subarachnoid CSF through the midline foramen in the roof of the fourth ventricle which now bears his name. He considered that CSF was formed both within the ventricular system from the choroid plexuses and outside the brain from the pia mater on the brain surface, and that there was an ebb-and-flow relationship between the intra- and extra-cerebral CSF compartments. He noted respiratory and cardiac pulsations in the CSF and considered that the function of the fluid was primarily to protect the brain and to float it within the skull. Luschka described the openings of the lateral recesses of the fourth ventricle in 1854 and 1855, and these anatomical features of the CSF in humans were confirmed by the extensive studies of Key and Retzius in 1875.

Hydrocephalus was recognised as a clinical entity (consisting of an excess of fluid within the cranial cavity) well before the time of Morgagni, but there was no understanding of its pathogenesis until after the end of the nineteenth century, and Morgagni's phrase 'hydrops cerebri' is an adequate account of the condition until the early 1900s.

The contributions made to the knowledge of the CSF by Weed and Dandy in the second decade of this century have had a fundamental influence upon subsequent views of spina bifida and hydrocephalus. On the basis of experiments in which potassium ferricyanide solution was injected into the ventricular system of pig embryos, Weed (1917) concluded that the roof of the rhombencephalon became permeable to the ferricyanide at the time of development of the choroid plexuses. From the appearance of the thin rhombencephalic roof, both in the developing pig and in human embryos, he concluded that continuity between the ventricular system and the extra-cerebral subarachnoid space was established by the secretory pressure of the CSF bursting through the roof of the rhombencephalon, thus forming the midline foramen. Weed's further observations on CSF production, the pathway of flow, and the sites of absorption into the venous system (1922) have become classical, and his interpretation of the embryological development and morphogenesis of the CSF pathway are now generally accepted (Weed 1938).

The work of Dandy and Blackfan (1913, 1914, 1917) and subsequent observations by Dandy (1918, 1919, 1922) established that hydrocephalus was caused by obstruction of the internal or external CSF pathways, or by occlusion of the foramina in the roof of the fourth ventricle connecting these compartments, and could be treated by removal of the choroid plexus or by removing or by-passing the obstruction. The now classical view of the CSF pathway of flow was presented succinctly by Cushing in 1926, under the title 'The Third Circulation and Its Channels' (Fig. 2.1).

These concepts eliminated the previously held views that hydrocephalus was primary (or idiopathic), and from 1920 onwards it became a matter of demonstrating the anatomical obstruction which caused the hydrocephalus. The well-established association between spina bifida and hydrocephalus underwent a reappraisal, and the concept that the excess of fluid within the neuraxis in some way caused the spina bifida malformation was reversed; it became a matter of explaining how the malformation obstructed the CSF pathway and caused the hydrocephalus.

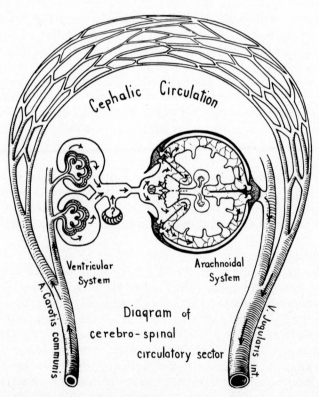

Fig. 2.1. Diagram of cerebro-spinal circulatory sector. (From Cushing 1926.) On the left the lateral and third ventricles are pictured as producing CSF from the choroid plexuses which are supplied by branches of the carotid artery. On the right the ventricular system and subarachnoid space are pictured as transferring CSF to the various systems via the sagittal sinus; the CSF flow (or third circulation) is pictured as within the cerebral circulation.

16

Current Concepts of CSF Embryology

The temporal relationship between posterior neuropore closure (at the 28-day stage) and the appearance of the choroid plexuses (at the seven-week stage) has been well established in many studies of human embryology (Hamilton *et al.* 1952, Schaltenbrand 1955, Bartelmez and Dekaban 1962, Brocklehurst 1968*a*), but the appearance of the midline foramen in the roof of the fourth ventricle has been variously reported. Waterston, in 1923, demonstrated the presence of the foramen in a 26mm embryo (seven and a half weeks), but most authorities have accepted that it appears in the third or fourth month of development (Wilson 1936, Schaltenbrand 1955, van Hoytema and van den Berg 1966). Recent investigations have shown the foramen to be present in the eighth week, and its appearance to be accompanied by staining of the surrounding cells with Periodic Acid Schiff reagent which indicates their glycogen content and can be taken as evidence of increased metabolic activity. These appearances can be interpreted as an active developmental process under genetic control rather than passive disruption of the roof of the fourth ventricle as suggested by Weed (Brocklehurst 1969*b*).

The relationship of the early stages of neural tube development to its contained fluid has been most fully studied in chick embryos. Cohen and Davies (1937), using a refined form of Weed's technique of potassium ferricyanide injection, showed that the injected fluid first escaped through the superior area of the roof of the rhomben-cephalon at the seventh day of development and then through the inferior area at the eighth and ninth days. They noted that the choroid plexuses of the third and lateral ventricles were formed at the seventh day, and that those of the fourth ventricle were formed at the eighth and ninth days. However, when Cohen and Davies (1938) repeated the same experiments in developing mammals, they found that the inferior medullary area remained intact and impermeable to the solution well after the time of formation of the choroid plexuses.

More recently, Jeliňek and Pexieder (1968, 1970) have studied the pressure of the fluid within the neural canal of the chick embryo and have found that it rises between the second (closure of the neuropore) and sixth day of incubation in a consistent manner. On the sixth day of incubation the single layer of neurectodermal cells which constitutes the roof of the rhombencephalon begins to separate and so permits the CSF to enter the mesenchyme of the future leptomeninges. They also showed that between the second and sixth day the fluid within the neural tube was produced by secretion of specialised neuroepithelial cells, and the pressure curve was built up prior to the appearance of the choroid plexuses. This development of pressure within the neural tube appears to be of importance in the formation of the cerebral vesicles in the chick, and these become deformed if the fluid escapes through a caudal myeloschisis. Their observations confirm the close temporal relationship between the development of the choroid plexus and the metapore in the roof of the fourth ventricle, but do not specifically confirm Weed's hypothesis. The pressure readings and the drop of pressure on the sixth day are compatible with the escape of fluid through the rhombencephalic roof as a result of the development of the foramen, rather than being the actual cause of this foramen. These recent observations upon the developing neural tube in the chick agree closely with those of Brocklehurst (1969*b*) in the human.

Hydrodynamic Concepts

From the time of Morgagni and Chiari onwards, the view that the spina bifida lesion and the brainstem malformation are in some way caused by an increased pressure of fluid within the developing neural tube has been widely held (*see* Chapter 1).

In 1932, van Houweninge Graftdijk demonstrated the valvular action of the brainstem malformation in spina bifida: the sac of the spinal lesion is often flat at birth and gradually distends during the neonatal period so that fluid is quite readily expressed from the sac upwards into the head (*i.e.* into the ventricles); the fontanelle pressure increases accordingly, but the fluid does not pass in the reverse direction when the fontanelle is compressed. This indicates that with pressure from above, the hindbrain malformation fits more firmly into the foramen magnum and further obstruction occurs at either the fourth ventricle or aqueduct level. When expressed upwards from below, the CSF floats up the brainstem and unplugs this obstruction. This clearly demonstrable phenomenon has been interpreted as indicating the way in which the brainstem malformation might have developed. For instance, after a detailed study of the pathology of 26 cases with open spina bifida lesions, Cameron (1957) concluded that the myeloschisis or meningocele lesion associated with spina bifida was a primary malformation and that this permitted a leak of cerebrospinal fluid from out of the neural tube into the amniotic cavity; thus the pressure required to develop the foramina in the roof of the fourth ventricle did not occur, and instead, a hindbrain malformation resulted.

Gardner (1965, 1966, 1968) went a little further and assumed that there is some unknown cause of a primary maldevelopment in the roof of the rhombencephalon which prevents the ventricular CSF from establishing the normal communication with the subarachnoid CSF, as postulated by Weed. An abnormal pressure develops within the primitive ventricles and central canal of the spinal cord, and this is decompressed by a bursting open of the caudal end of the developing neural tube to form a myeloschisis and an accompanying spina bifida. It is important to recognise that this hypothesis must assume that the secretory pressure is built up by the activity of the neuroepithelium itself, for the appearance of a myeloschisis in an 8mm human embryo described by Patten (1953) and the 5mm specimen described by Lemire *et al.* (1965) both established the occurrence of this malformation at the stage in embryological development between posterior neuropore closure and the appearance of the choroid plexuses. These examples resemble the condition termed 'hydrops cerebri et medullaris' by Morgagni rather than hydrocephalus as understood in the classical terms of Weed and Dandy. It should also be noted that the histological appearances in both of these embryos were those of increased tissue at the level of the myeloschisis rather than the kind of attenuation which would be expected to accompany a bursting of the neural tube.

In recent extensive reviews of human embryonic material Padget concluded that the blebs which she observed in association with myeloschitic lesions were the probable cause of these lesions, and were in themselves evidence of a ruptured neural tube (Padget 1968, 1970). She related these blebs to clefts which occurred in specimens with intact neural tubes, and concluded that these had been through the stage of what she termed 'neuroschisis' and had healed. However, Lendon (1968*a*)

18

studied the same kind of lesions which he noted in the embryogenesis of spina bifida produced experimentally in rats, and observed that the blebs and haematomata occurred not only directly beneath areas of terminal myeloschisis but also alongside the lesions in a paramedian position, and sometimes quite rostral to the lesion. He suggested that both the phenomena and the spina bifida lesion were evidence of the damage caused by the teratogenic action of the Trypan blue, and were not in themselves the actual mechanism whereby the neural tube was disrupted.

These hypothetical concepts of the hydrodynamics of spina bifida and hydrocephalus are even more unsatisfactory when the actual pathology of the fetal and newborn spina bifida specimens are studied: extensive hydrocephalus associated with myeloschisis and no communication between the abnormal fourth ventricle and the central canal of the spinal cord has been well described from the time of Cleland onwards, and there is sometimes no connection between the central canal and the surface of the myeloschisis (Brocklehurst 1968a, 1969a, 1971).

Current Concepts of CSF Morphology, Physiology and Pathology

The comparative morphology of the CSF has hardly been explored. Recent incursions into the field indicate that there are many vertebrates early in the evolutionary scale in which there is no direct connection between the intracerebral and extracerebral spinal fluid: in many fishes the hydraulic functions of the extracerebral CSF appear to be replaced by a large subdural fluid space. Vertebrates higher up the evolutionary scale develop lateral foramina in the roof of the fourth ventricle, which appear not to be directly related to the development of the choroid plexuses in these species. Only in some of the Old World Monkeys and anthropoids is a foramen of Magendie present which is similar to that in man.

Little is known of the dynamics of the CSF space during intra-uterine development in the human, but it is well known that late fetal and neonatal specimens of extensive spina bifida have accompanying hydrocephalus (as evidenced by dilatation of the lateral and third ventricles). The obvious obstructions to the CSF pathway, which can be seen in the aqueduct, the deformed fourth ventricle, and the foramen magnum (occupied by the malformed brainstem), are assumed to be the cause of the hydrocephalus. This view is in keeping with the classical concepts of obstructive hydrocephalus promoted by Dandy.

Russell and Donald (1935) were the first observers to conclude that the malformed brainstem was the site of the obstruction, which view was partly supported by the observations of Ingraham and Scott (1943) and those of Cameron (1957). Obstruction to the CSF pathway at the level of the aqueduct is variously reported and appears to depend upon the circumstances in which the study is made: it is not a common lesion in fetal studies, although it has been reported as a primary lesion appearing prior to hydrocephalus in some teratogenic experiments (Warkany 1971). Alvord (1961) reviewed this subject extensively and considered that aqueduct obstruction was present in 50 per cent of spina bifida cases, but Emery, in a more recent study (1974, see Chapter 3), found deformities in all of a 100 cases. Emery concluded, from the appearances of the deformities, that the aqueduct became shortened in length and compressed from side to side as a secondary phenomenon in development, and periaqueductal gliosis and adhesions of the ependyma (to produce the appearance called 'forking' of the aqueduct) followed from this process. Williams (1973) has put forward the hypothesis that the so-called 'aqueduct stenosis' is indeed secondary to hydrocephalus, through a process of lateral compression from the distended lateral ventricles: observations of its increasing frequency in spina bifida from the earliest embryonic periods onwards are compatible with this view.

Assuming the brainstem malformation itself constitutes the obstruction, in the classical sense, to bulk-flow of CSF, and that this exists for at least the last three months of intra-uterine development (if not earlier), then a more profound degree of ventricular dilatation would be expected than that found in the neonatal spina bifida patient. It could be concluded that during these months CSF production and absorption occurs independently of bulk-flow through the classical pathway. A CSF system in which there is no communication between the ventricles and the sub-arachnoid space reproduces the state which is natural for some simpler animals, and it is possible, in this situation, that absorption of CSF from the ventricular system occurs directly across the ependymal lining.

The independent rôle of the extracerebral (subarachnoid) CSF in humans is illustrated by the observation of a fully developed CSF-containing subarachnoid space in the neonatal spina bifida infant (during shunting procedures), where there can have been no continuity between internal and external cerebrospinal fluid for a very long period of time, if ever (Brocklehurst 1974b). These concepts have also been emphasised by Milhorat et al. (1971) and Milhorat (1972), who have demonstrated the independency of the subarachnoid space from bulk-flow out of the ventricular system.

Experiments performed by Dandy have been repeated with more modern techniques. Bering (1962) demonstrated that ventricular dilatation in experimental hydrocephalus depended upon the pulsation of the choroid plexus rather than just upon the obstruction of the ventricular system. Milhorat and Mosher (1970) also demonstrated that hydrocephalus could occur without the choroid plexuses, and this was taken as indicating an extra-choroid plexus source of cerebrospinal fluid that produced some kind of pressure differential in the obstructed ventricular system. All of these recent observations require a reappraisal of CSF morphology, physiology and pathology, and also some modification of the bulk-flow pattern laid down in the classical work of Weed and Dandy. Bulk-flow, as shown by isotope studies, is a relatively slow phenomenon, and probably not the only determinant of pressure within the ventricular system.

It follows from these observations that the views of the pathogenesis of spina bifida and its related hydrocephalus which are based upon these classical concepts are by no means so tenable in the light of current knowledge.

A Present Day View of Spina Bifida and Hydrocephalus

It is of basic importance to recognise that the group of congenital malformations that have in common the separation of the vertebral elements in the midline (which we can call 'spina bifida') covers a wide spectrum, from such conditions as spina bifida occulta with minimal neurological involvement, to gross spinal rachischisis with anencephaly. The variety of phenomena associated with spina bifida, such as mesodermal malformations, heterotopias, duplications, teratomatous malformations and dysplasias, suggest a process of disturbed embryogenesis in various directions rather than a single hydrodynamic phenomenon.

Genetic studies of spina bifida patients (see Chapter 5) reveal no more than a 'polygenically-inherited predisposition', and since experimental teratology can reproduce the condition, the likelihood is that it is caused by some environmental factor which may or may not be specific, acting upon a genetically-susceptible embryo at around the 28-day stage. The teratological phenomena so produced may disturb the developing embryo in a number of different ways, and may affect a number of different embryological processes (see Table 2.I). These disturbances in embryonic development are presumably the result of abnormal DNA patterns operating through 'messenger RNA' upon cellular metabolism and development. The individual pattern which occurs may depend upon the exact time of action of the teratogenetic insult; acting in relationship to anterior neuropore closure, anencephaly will occur, and the various degrees of myeloschisis and the lesions associated with spina bifida will occur if the teratogenic action is just before or around the time of posterior neuropore closure. On the whole, the more extensive lesions involving the thoracic and thoraco-lumbar spinal cord are associated with a greater degree of cerebral malformations and accompanying mesodermal malformations. This concept gives a point of origin for considering the pathogenesis of spina bifida, but leaves the aetiology of the condition unknown at present.

The structural abnormalities are established by about the 28th day of development, and the manifestations of these occur within the basic developmental pattern of the central nervous system and its surrounding mesoderm: in addition, secondary mechanical and hydrodynamic forces produce further deformities *in utero*. In the majority of cases, *i.e.* where the primary abnormality of neural tube closure is so severe that the neural tube actually remains open and there is a skin defect obvious at birth (see Chapter 3), the associated malformation of the brainstem consists of encephalocranial disproportion. At some stage, presumably in later intra-uterine development, CSF fluid bulk-flow is obstructed by the brainstem malformation, and the increased intraventricular pressure results in dilatation of the ventricles and subsequent dilatation of the cranial vault. Lesions of the aqueduct may be further superimposed upon this by secondary distortion and compression, and the pathology of the neonatal infant with spina bifida is established.

At birth there is increased bulk-flow and the hydrocephalus becomes more apparent; enlargement of the soft cranial vault becomes rapid.

Associated with the abnormalities of the structures derived directly from the neural tube are abnormalities of the adjacent mesoderm. These are manifested in the structure of the cranial vault, vertebrae and ribs (see Chapter 3). There is some overlap of these teratological phenomena with other conditions such as encephaloceles, congenital lower limb abnormalities (including sympodia) and other neural crest abnormalities such as von Recklinghausen's neurofibromatosis (see Chapter 3).

The further course of the disease involves continued secondary deformities of mesodermal and neurectodermal structures. Progressive hydrocephalus tends to

TABLE 2.I.
Teratological processes—as illustrated by spina bifida

PRIMARY PROCESSES	
Developmental arrest	
ectoderm	skin defects (spina bifida aperta)
neurectoderm	myeloschisis
mesoderm	bifid vertebrae (spina bifida)
Heterotopia (normal tissue in abnormal places)	
ectoderm	hypertrichosis, pigmentation
neurectoderm	cerebral and cerebellar heterotopias
mesoderm	lipomatous masses/nephroic tubules in spina bifida lesion
Duplications	
ectoderm	cutaneous appendages over spina bifida
neurectoderm	diplomyelia, diastematomyelia
mesoderm	double vertebrae, double ribs, duplication of ureters and kidneys
endoderm	intestinal cysts, duplications (with ventral spina bifida)
Dysplasia	
ectoderm	dysplastic dermis over meningocele
neurectoderm	myelodysplasia, hydromyelia, Cleland-Arnold-Chiari malformation
mesoderm	dysplastic vertebrae, ribs, skull
Neoplasia	
ectoderm	teratomatous malformation
neurectoderm	ditto
mesoderm	ditto
endoderm	ditto
Disproportions	
ectoderm	encephalo-cranial/myelo-vertebral disproportion
neurectoderm	ditto
mesoderm	ditto

SECONDARY PROCESSES	
Hydrodynamic	hydrocephalus (aqueduct stenosis)
Mechanical	talipes, kyphosis, scoliosis
Degenerative	neural plaque degeneration

reach an arrest dependent upon the size of the meningocele sac and the size of the ultimate ventricular dilatation.

This view of the nature of spina bifida places the emphasis upon teratogenesis and away from some of the earlier hydrodynamic concepts. The possible relationship between the teratogenetic action and the fluid content of the early neural tube at the crucial moment of posterior neuropore closure remains to be determined.

CHAPTER 3

The Pathology of Spina Bifida
and the Associated Hydrocephalus

Nomenclature

The introduction, in Chapter 1, of a number of terms within their historical context indicates the complexity of this subject. Some of the earlier terms are generalised descriptions which have remained clinically useful, and the later ones have been added to amplify the detailed pathology and possible pathogenesis. Duplication of descriptive terms by the use of words derived separately from both Greek and Latin languages has added to the confusion, and there is now need of some simplification. Etymological accuracy is valuable in describing the detailed pathology of a condition, but some compromise with the practical usefulness of words which have proved clinically valuable must be achieved, and, as Humpty Dumpty pointed out to Alice, we have the right to make words mean what we want them to mean.

Tables 3.I and 3.II represent a generally acceptable classification of the spinal and cranial lesions, and in elaborating these terms the synonyms will be mentioned.

General Terms
Spina bifida

This remains the most useful general term and is derived from the original description by Tulp (see Chapter 1) of an infant with a spina (dorsi) bifida lesion. It describes the separation of the vertebral elements in the midline which is the common feature of a whole range of conditions, and since the vast majority of these are lesions of the dorsal elements of the vertebrae, we do not usually add the genitive noun, but rather specify the rarer spina ventralis bifida when discussing the condition in which the vertebral body itself is separated into two halves by a cleft.

Spinal dysraphism

This is also a good general term derived from Greek roots and meaning a disturbance of the formation of a tissue junction line, in this case viewing the spine as a raphé (the term 'status dysraphicus' is etymologically unsatisfactory and a bit too general to be useful). Spinal dysraphism has the advantage of not implying any particular pathogenesis in the disturbance of the midline structures, but it seems a somewhat inadequate term for the complexity of the spinal column and neural tube when compared with raphés elsewhere in the body.

Rachischisis

This is a term, again of Greek origin, used by a number of authors to describe the split spine. As such, it has no particular advantage over 'spina bifida', and etymologically, there is a slight suggestion that the suffix means splitting of an already formed structure, which is a view of the pathogenesis of spina bifida not fully acceptable. On the other hand the term has been applied in medicine to anything which has the appearance of a split, without too much regard to the actual pathogenesis, and as such the useful term 'myeloschisis' has been retained in this account to describe the very basic lesion in the spinal cord.

-Cele and -coele

In describing the pathological lesions associated with spina bifida, these suffixes are frequently used and have given rise to some difficulty. '-Cele' is derived from the Greek 'kele', which means a hernia, and as such has a connotation which is less satisfactory when applied to the congenital malformations of the neural canal than to other pathological conditions. '-Coele' is derived from the Greek 'koilia' meaning a cavity, which is purely descriptive, and in many ways more acceptable. The westernisation of spelling, however, has caused the diphthong to be dropped from the suffix '-coele' and this is now commonly spelt '-cele', so that the etymological derivation is no longer clear. Such ambiguity is non-committal but a bit unsatisfactory.

Spina Bifida Aperta (see Fig. 3.1, *a* to *f*)

The ectodermal derivatives over clinically significant spina bifida are nearly always abnormal; the commonest appearance is that of completely deficient skin with exposure of the neural tissue and open spinal canal. *Spina bifida aperta* is the correct term for this open lesion, seen most clearly in the newborn with extensive thoraco-lumbar spina bifida. In other cases the spina bifida lesion is covered by a poorly epithelialised membrane, which, with the passage of time, becomes more tensely cystic and more completely epithelialised. This type of lesion justifies the term *spina bifida cystica* used in the earlier literature: any spina bifida lesion which is obvious from inspection of the abnormal overlying ectoderm can be termed *spina bifida manifesta,* which is slightly less specific than spina bifida aperta. In this account, the large group of spina bifida lesions over which the skin is incompletely epithelialised will be termed *spina bifida aperta,* since this indicates that the lesion is potentially open to infection and is an important distinction in clinical management. The terms 'manifesta' and 'cystica' will be dispensed with.

Spina Bifida Occulta

This is the appropriate term to use when epithelialised skin covers the spina bifida lesion and it is more or less hidden. X-rays of the lumbar spine frequently reveal minor degrees of spina bifida occulta affecting the lower lumbar or upper sacral vertebrae in otherwise normal persons, although these lesions may be of no neurological significance and may be covered by normal skin. The spina bifida occulta cases of more importance are those over which the skin often bears an abnormal tuft of hair or is dimpled, pigmented, or prominent, due to a subcutaneous lipomatous mass. Occasionally the ectodermal abnormality is a so-called 'dermal sinus' which runs from the skin down as far as the bifid vertebrae, or even into the dura. To the unwary clinician this is indeed an occult lesion, but in fact it runs the same risk of intraspinal infection as the more common spina bifida aperta. (See Ch. 7 and Figs. 7.1, 7.2.)

TABLE 3.I

Spinal lesions in spina bifida (aperta et occulta)

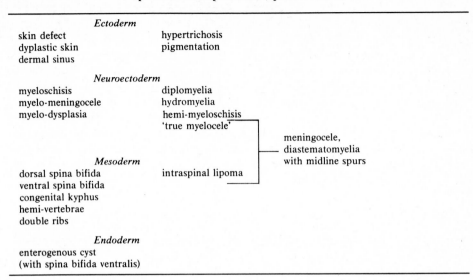

Ectoderm

skin defect	hypertrichosis
dyplastic skin	pigmentation
dermal sinus	

Neuroectoderm

myeloschisis   diplomyelia
myelo-meningocele   hydromyelia
myelo-dysplasia   hemi-myeloschisis
'true myelocele'

    meningocele,
    diastematomyelia
    with midline spurs

Mesoderm

dorsal spina bifida   intraspinal lipoma
ventral spina bifida
congenital kyphus
hemi-vertebrae
double ribs

Endoderm

enterogenous cyst
(with spina bifida ventralis)

TABLE 3.II

Cranial lesions in spina bifida

	Hindbrain	*Midbrain*	*Forebrain*
Neurectoderm Cleland- Arnold- Chiari malformation	Caudal prolongation of cerebellar vermis Caudal displacement of flattened fourth ventricle Caudal displacement of dorsally-kinked medulla	Tectal beaking Aqueduct stenosis	Micropolygyria Enlarged massa intermedia
Mesoderm	Craniolacunae Enlarged foramen magnum Eversion of petrous temporal bones 'Keyhole' anterior fontanelle	Narrow falx cerebri Low-attached tentorium cerebelli Enlarged tentorial hiatus	Elongated vein of Galen Short straight sinus, low-lying torcula Caudally displaced vertebro-basilar arteries

Lesions of the Neural Tube (see Figs. 3.1, *a* to *f*, and 3.2, 3.3, 3.5, 3.6, 3.7)
Myeloschisis (Fig. 3.1*a*)

This is the wide-open neural tube seen in the common thoraco-lumbar spina bifida aperta examined within a few hours of birth. Viewed dorsally, it can be likened to an anchovy fillet in appearance: the open central canal constitutes a median furrow and the embryonic sulcus limitans makes paramedian furrows which mark out the alar and basal laminae. The nerve roots which leave the ventral aspect of this 'neural plaque' proceed to their respective foramina; the upper ones directed cephalad, the middle transversely, and the lower ones caudad.

In cross section the lesion is surmounted by degenerated ependymal epithelium in the centre and consists of a mass of dorsally placed grey matter containing neurones grouped centrally and laterally, and a mass of ventrally placed white matter consisting of segmental and intersegmental tracts symmetrically distorted (Figs. 3.2, 3.3).

Myelomeningocele (Fig. 3.1*b*)

This term has a clinical usage so widespread that it is almost synonymous with spina bifida aperta. Etymologically, it is most satisfactorily interpreted as meaning a cystic lesion of the meninges around the malformed neural tube. It describes very well that group of infants born with a cystic lesion (in the lumbar or sacral region) consisting of a multiloculated cavity which is lined by membranes continuous with the arachnoid around the spinal cord, and containing fluid more or less in continuity with the CSF. This arachnoidal membrane is covered ventrolaterally by tissue continuous with the spinal dura as far as the level of the ectoderm, and dorsilaterally the ectoderm itself encroaches upon the sac around the base to form a poorly epithelialised contribution to the membranes. In the centre of the lesion there is usually external evidence of the abnormal neural tissue surmounted by granulation tissue and consisting of a mass of gliosis and nerve fibres replacing part of the conus medullaris of the spinal cord. The membrane most immediately surrounding this type of plaque is the thickened derivative of the arachnoid. The spinal cord can usually be traced coming from the spinal canal into the upper end of the myelomeningocele sac, even when this is situated in the sacral region; *i.e.* the spinal cord remains relatively elongated in these lesions. Very rarely, the myelomeningocele sac consists of an arachnoidal cavity in which there are only aberrant nerve fibres derived from the cauda equina.

Myelocele

This is a rather unsatisfactory term, whatever its assumed etymology. On the one hand it suggests a herniation of the spinal cord, which is not an accurate description, and on the other hand that the cavity is actually within the spinal cord (myelocoele), which again is not the pathology of the spinal cord lesion as it presents in the common spina bifida aperta.

Myelodysplasia (Fig. 3.1*d*)

This is a useful term which describes satisfactorily that disturbance in the formation of the spinal cord which consists of a more or less symmetrical glial proliferation and mal-alignment of the white matter in the region of the conus medullaris; this is often seen not only in myelomeningocele lesions but also in spina bifida occulta lesions.

Meningocele (Fig. 3.1c)

In this condition the cystic lesion (which is apparent by inspection or dissection) consists of meninges only and contains fluid in continuity with the CSF, but no neural tissue. It is relatively rare among spina bifida aperta lesions, and, when it exists, there may still be an associated dysplasia of the neural tube derivatives lying within the spinal canal and beneath the neck of the meningocele. The meningeal layers involved in the meningocele are derivatives of the arachnoid and the fibrous dura.

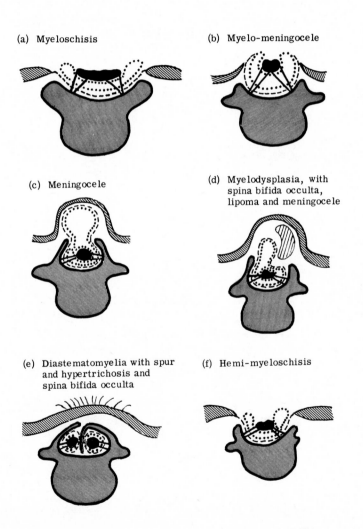

(a) Myeloschisis

(b) Myelo-meningocele

(c) Meningocele

(d) Myelodysplasia, with spina bifida occulta, lipoma and meningocele

(e) Diastematomyelia with spur and hypertrichosis and spina bifida occulta

(f) Hemi-myeloschisis

Fig. 3.1. Cross section diagrams of spinal lesions in spina bifida.

Diplomyelia

This is a lesion in which the spinal cord is actually duplicated along part of its length, the two cords being complete with appropriate ventral and dorsal horns and central canal. It is a relatively rare lesion in such complete form, and has been described both above and below the site of the spina bifida aperta, the duplication being usually side by side but occasionally antero-posterior. It can be considered a more extreme form of diastematomyelia.

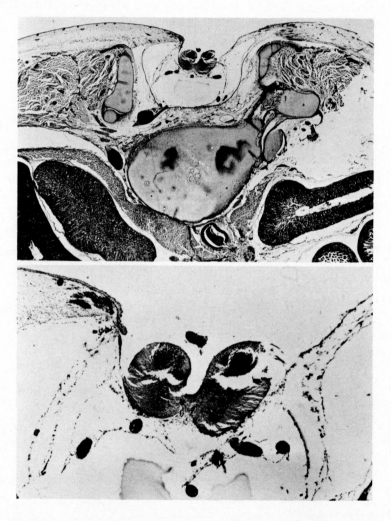

Fig. 3.2 (*top*). Transverse section of 95mm spina bifida fetus at level of myeloschisis (× 20). The myeloschisis lies exposed and fragmented in the upper part of the section.

Fig. 3.3 (*bottom*). Myeloschis (detail from Fig. 3.2).

28

Diastematomyelia (Fig. 3.1*e*)

In this condition, the spinal cord is split into two halves along the sagittal plane, each half having at least one dorsal and one ventral horn. The central canal is more or less completely formed in each half and there are rudimentary horns in the paramedian grey matter. The split in the spinal cord is usually accompanied by a strand of fibrous tissue running from the dorsal to the ventral dura, and in some cases the dura in the midline encircles a bony spur which is attached to one of the laminae of a spina bifida lesion dorsally, and to the dorsal aspect of the vertebral body ventrally. The diastematomyelia with bony spur is a not uncommon accompaniment of a spina bifida occulta lesion which is covered by skin bearing a tuft of hair (hypertrichosis). (See Figs. 3.6 and 3.7.)

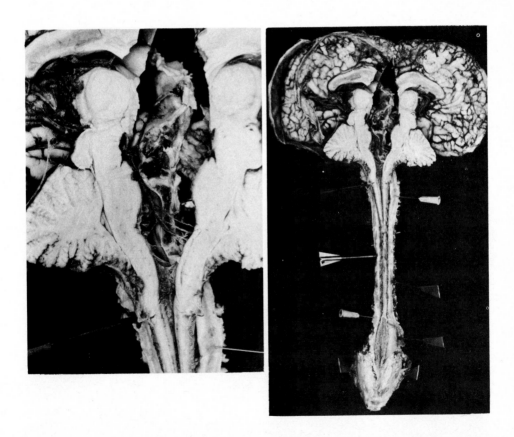

Fig. 3.4 (*left*). Cleland-Arnold-Chiari malformation, sagittally sectioned (detail from Fig. 3.5).
Fig. 3.5 (*right*). Full dissection of lumbo-sacral spina bifida specimen showing lumbo-sacral myeloschisis, transverse nerve roots and attenuated cord just rostral to plaque, caudally directed thoracic nerve roots, medullary 'knickung', caudal prolongation of cerebellar vermis, flattened fourth ventricle, tectal beaking, large massa intermedia, micro polygyria and hydrocephalus.

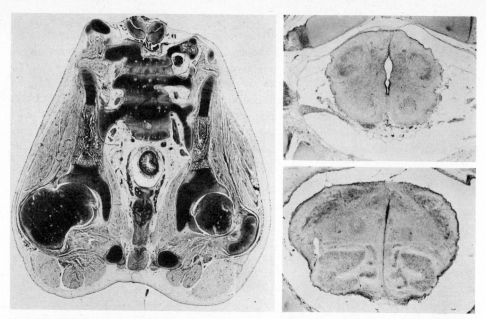

Fig. 3.6 (*left*). Diastematomyelia. Transverse section of tail bud at sacral level in 95mm fetus with thoraco-lumbar spina bifida (× 20).

Fig. 3.8 (*top right*). Hydromyelia (and syringomyelia). Transverse section of cervical spinal cord in 95mm spina bifida fetus with thoraco-lumbar spina bifida.

Fig. 3.9 (*bottom right*). Obliteration of central canal. Transverse section of 95mm fetus with thoraco-lumbar spina bifida.

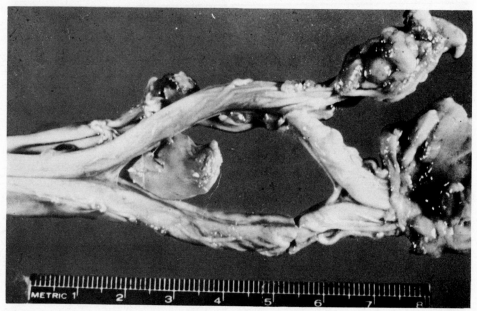

Fig. 3.7. Dissected specimen of diastematomyelia with spur.

Hydromyelia

This is a dilatation of the central canal still lined by ependyma and it may be found on the cephalic side of a spina bifida lesion. When the dilatation extends beyond the ependyma and is in continuity with a cavity lined by neural tissue, the lesion can be described as a 'syringomyelia'. Both of these lesions are frequently found in the spinal cord on the cephalic side of a spina bifida aperta lesion. Forking and blind termination of the central canal are also found, particularly in the cervical region just below the brainstem malformation (see Figs. 3.8, 3.9) (Cleland 1883, Brocklehurst 1969a, Mackenzie and Emery 1971).

The Cranial Lesions
The hindbrain malformation (Cleland-Arnold-Chiari malformation) (Fig. 3.4)

This malformation occurs to some degree in nearly all spina bifida aperta lesions and consists of the following:
(a) caudal prolongation of the cerebellar vermis, the degree varying from a bulging of the vermis right into the fourth ventricle and upper central canal, to an almost insignificant caudal projection (Groups 1 to 4, Schwalbe and Gredig 1907);
(b) the fourth ventricle is displaced into the upper cervical canal;
(c) the medulla is displaced into the upper cervical canal and usually has a dorsally directed kink or knuckle ('Knickung').
The historical origin of the eponyms for this brainstem malformation are fully described in Chapter 1.

In addition to these main features, the lower end of the fourth ventricle is often closed off from the central canal of the cervical spinal cord, and the site of the foramen of Magendie and inferior medullary velum is occupied by the distorted cerebellar vermis. The malformation fits closely into the enlarged foramen magnum of the skull and is surrounded by thickened arachnoid. The actual weight of the cerebellum in this malformation is less than that in the normal neonate (Variend and Emery 1973), and histologically, the central lobes of the cerebellum show chronic necrosis, loss of Purkinje cells, heterotopia and dysplasia. In the culmen and declive there are areas of acute necrosis (Variend and Emery 1974). Around the lower end of the brainstem malformation the meninges are thickened and there is evidence of chronic inflammation and venous infarction.

Midbrain malformations

The deformity of the colliculi of the midbrain (originally described by Cleland 1883) was reported in detail by Daniel and Strich (1958), who described the inferior colliculi at the apex of a beak-like deformity and the superior colliculi plastered down at the base ('tectal beaking'). (See Fig. 3.4.)

Deformities of the aqueduct have been variously reported in different series of studies on the pathology of spina bifida. The earlier accounts mention occasional atresia of the aqueduct (Russell and Donald 1935). More recent descriptions record narrowing of the aqueduct, with forking and periaqueductal gliosis in many cases. Emery (1974) has detailed the pathology in 100 cases of spina bifida examined post mortem and has found the structure blocked, shortened in length and angulated in

31

various fashions, with attachments of the adjacent areas of the ependyma giving macroscopic obliteration of the lumen. However, the duct is actually patent when examined histologically.

Forebrain abnormalities

In nearly all examples of spina bifida (with or without hydrocephalus) the cerebral gyri are small and increased in number, such that the normal recognised configurations of sulci are absent and the sulci which are present do not penetrate as deeply as in the normal brain (a condition known as micropolygyria). Dilatation of the lateral ventricles is the rule rather than the exception, and histological examination of the cerebral cortex reveals clusters of cells in abnormal position (cortical heterotopia). Other cerebral abnormalities associated with the brainstem mal-formations include the prolonged course of the cranial nerves VI to XII to reach their skull foramina, and the cephalad course of the upper two to three cervical nerves to reach their intervertebral foramina. In early cases there is a fusion of the thalamus in the forebrain to form a large massa intermedia which becomes attenuated with dilatation of the third ventricle consequent upon hydrocephalus.

Other Primary Lesions (Mesodermal Abnormalities)

Vertebral deformities

At the site of a spina bifida lesion, the pedicles of the vertebrae are everted and the interpedicular distance widened so that the spinal canal is relatively much larger; a situation which can be described as *myelo-vertebral disproportion*. There is a similar disproportion above the spina bifida lesion caused by narrowing or attenuation of a segment or two of the spinal cord, and in the upper cervical region the somewhat widened spinal canal is relatively crowded by the brainstem abnormality and upper cervical spinal cord.

The vertebral bodies are frequently mis-shapen, either in the antero-posterior direction, to form a congenital kyphus in the lumbar region, or in the lateral direction by wedge or hemivertebrae, giving rise to a gross congenital scoliosis often affecting segments above the spina bifida lesion.

Rib abnormalities

Bifurcation, duplication and absence of ribs is common in severe spina bifida cases. Other supporting tissues of mesodermal origin are often malformed; there is commonly an excess of lipomatous tissue occurring either within the spinal canal or subcutaneously at the site of the spina bifida occulta lesion, and this is sometimes so lobulated as to warrant the term 'lipoma' (Emery and Lendon 1969, see Fig. 3.1d). Rarely, derivatives of the mesonephros are found among the abnormal tissue at the spina bifida site.

Blood vessels

There is frequently a cluster of dilated arteries and veins lying on the surface of the neural plaque in the dysplastic cases; this was described in the older literature as *area vasculosa.* Blood vessels around the brainstem are abnormal, and in particular the vertebral and basilar arteries are caudally displaced, but not so far caudally displaced as the posterior inferior cerebellar arteries which are taken well down into the cervical spinal canal (Emery and Levick 1966). The superior sagittal sinus is sometimes duplicated, and parietal and occipital emissary veins are well developed. The internal cerebral veins are often deformed (Blaauw 1970).

Cranial vault
There are commonly defects in the membraneous bone of the cranial vault which are known as craniolacunae (Lückenschadel). With the passage of time these defects gradually ossify, regardless of whether or not the hydrocephalus is treated, and then the radiological appearance is often similar to that described as 'convolutional marking' associated with raised intracranial pressure in childhood or infancy. It is probable that the basic cause of these craniolacunae is a mesodermal dysplasia, and there is a high association of craniolacunae with severe brainstem malformation and hydrocephalus, and with subsequent mental retardation (Vogt and Wyatt 1941, McCoy *et al.* 1967).

Fontanelles and sutures
The anterior fontanelle is often extended well down into the metopic suture of the frontal bone. This gives the large key-hole appearance, which is a very characteristic dysplastic feature of the skull in spina bifida with hydrocephalus. In addition to this, the anterior fontanelle is enlarged, and often the lateral fontanelles at the asterion and pterion are large and membraneous. The lambdoidal and sagittal sutures are often widely separated, and this may be a valuable sign of hydrocephalus in infants with a globular skull that lacks the other dysplastic features already described.

Skull base
This is often grossly abnormal, with the posterior fossa very shallow, the attachment of the tentorium cerebelli low, the foramen magnum large, the jugular foramina enlarged, the petrous temporal bones flattened and the basal angle increased (Kruyff and Jeffs 1966).

Meninges and venous sinuses
The hiatus of the tentorium cerebelli is enlarged and the straight sinus shortened as it runs to the inferiorly placed torcula of the sinuses. Consequently, the great cerebral vein of Galen is elongated. The falx cerebri in spina bifida is nearly always relatively shallow.
Primary renal abnormalities, *e.g.* agenesis of the kidneys, hypoplasia of the kidneys and abnormalities of the ureters are significantly frequent in spina bifida patients, quite apart from the secondary abnormalities of the renal tract which result from the abnormal co-ordination of bladder sphincters with detrusor muscle contraction (see Chapter 11).

Rarer Varieties of Lesions Associated with Spina Bifida

Hemi-myelocele (see Fig. 3.1*f*).

This was the term given by Duckworth *et al.* (1968) to an asymmetrical myeloschisis in the lumbar region: one half of the cord is almost fully formed and the other half severely dysplastic and with abnormal roots. Associated with this there is asymmetrical development of the underlying vertebral bodies, with the shortening of these vertebral bodies on the dysplastic side forming the concavity of a very severe scoliosis. The lower limb on the dysplastic side is paralysed, while the limb on the other side has relatively normal neurological function.

Double myelomeningocele

This is found at the rate of one to two per cent in any extensive series of spina bifida aperta patients. It consists of a lower lesion which is usually a frank myeloschisis in the thoraco-lumbar region, normal intervening skin, and then an upper limited spina bifida aperta with underlying myeloschisis. The level of the neurological lesion, however, is referable to the uppermost of the two lesions, and the condition represents a serious and extensive malformation.

'True myelocele'

This is an uncommon lesion which occurs in the upper thoracic or cervical region. A meningocele sac filled by a nodule of glial tissue extends from the dorsal aspect of the spinal cord (which lies in the spinal canal beneath the spina bifida). The nodule of glial tissue contains a diverticulum of the central canal, and could therefore be described as a myelocele, *i.e.* in the sense of a cavity within the spinal cord. The nodule of tissue is non-functional and can be excised without impairing spinal cord nerve function, provided that it is not removed below the neck of the sac.

Spina bifida ventralis

The ventral spina bifida lesion usually occurs in the bodies of the upper thoracic or lower cervical vertebrae, and the cleft is often associated with an enterogenous cyst. It has been suggested that the embryogenesis of the lesion is a persistence of the transitory neurenteric canal and that the condensing mesoderm then splits around this.

Teratological Overlaps

In addition to this wide spectrum of lesions associated with spina bifida, there is the occasional occurrence of an overlap between this condition and other congenital malformations, *e.g.* spina bifida ventralis and co-existent enterogenous cyst. There have, too, been cases in which a teratomatous malformation (consisting of derivatives of endoderm and mesoderm) extends dorsally into the spina bifida sac splitting the myeloschisis, and ventrally into the peritoneal cavity through a ventral spina bifida (Brocklehurst, unpublished). Neurofibromatosis (an abnormality of neural crest derivatives) has been described in association with spina bifida, and there is clearly some overlap between sacral spina bifida, sacral agenesis and the ano-coccygeal teratoma. The extreme tail-bud malformation is exemplified by Arnold's original case of severe spina bifida with sympodia.

Developmental Pathology of Spinal Lesions

Disturbances of the early development of the neural tube by various teratological processes were described and discussed in Chapters 1 and 2. This section is concerned with the further development of the spinal lesion which results in the variety of findings in the neonatal infant with spina bifida.

Closure of the posterior neuropore occurs in the lumbar region of the spine. Holmdahl (1925) thought that it occurred opposite the fourth or fifth lumbar segments, and Barson (1970a), quoting Arey (1954), considered that it occurred between the first and second lumbar vertebrae (25-somite stage) (see also Hamilton *et al*. 1952 and Chapter 1).

All the segments caudal to the site of posterior neuropore closure are formed from the tail-bud process. Barson correlated the distribution of the sites of the spina bifida lesion by clinical and radiological surveys, and concluded that when the first lumbar segment was involved then the whole of the tail-bud process was disturbed and a spina bifida extending down into the sacrum occurred. Thus, all the high lumbar and thoraco-lumbar lesions are in fact thoraco-lumbar sacral as far as the bifid vertebrae are concerned, although the more caudal parts of the lesion are often covered by complete ectoderm. On the other hand, lesions occurring in the lower lumbar region or sacral region are more limited in extent and also in depth. In any large series of spina bifida patients, about 50 per cent of the lesions involve L1 or higher, and can be described primarily as thoraco-lumbar. About twenty-five per cent of the lesions are lumbo-sacral, and the remainder consist of sacral and (more rarely) limited thoracic and cervical lesions.

After the establishment of the neural tube defect there is a disturbance in the normal reationship between the spinal cord segments and the vertebrae. Normally, the conus medullaris undergoes a relatively rapid ascent to the level of the fourth lumbar vertebra by the 19th week of pregnancy, and thereafter ascends more slowly to end approximately opposite the lower border of the second lumbar vertebra at full-term. It attains the accepted adult level of the first lumbar vertebra by about two months post-natally (Barson 1970b).

When there is a full myeloschisis associated with a spina bifida lesion, the neural plaque remains at its initial segmental level and the nerves from the middle of the plaque proceed directly laterally to their exit foramina. The nerves from the upper part of the plaque proceed in a slightly cephalic direction and the nerves of the spinal cord segments immediately on the cephalic side of the myeloschisis proceed in a more caudal direction. The nerve roots from higher spinal segments achieve their normal caudal direction to their exit foramina, and the course of the spinal nerves only becomes abnormal again when the upper cervical segments are surmounted by the brainstem malformation and are caudally displaced so that the roots proceed in a more cephalad direction. These features are well illustrated in the dissected specimen in Fig. 3.5.

Quantitative examination of the spinal cord segments in fetal specimens with spina bifida shows an increased amount of tissue at the level of the myeloschisis, a relatively narrow cord in the segments just on the cephalic side of the lesion, and relatively normal size of cord segments above this (Barry *et al*. 1957; Brocklehurst

1968*a*, 1969*a*). The studies by Emery and Naik (1968) and Naik and Emery (1968) of post-natal spina bifida cases have shown that the segments just cephalad to the neural plaque are elongated, and the upper cervical segments just below the brainstem malformation are abnormally shortened.

Lendon (1968*b*, 1969) has studied the neurone population at various levels in spinal cords with spina bifida lesions. He found that at the level of the neural plaque the neurone population was reduced in proportion to the degree of dysplasia or full myeloschisis. When allowance was made for the segmental lengths on the cephalic side of the myeloschisis, the neurone population was calculated as normal, but in the upper thoracic and cervical regions there was some reduction in the population when hydromyelia or syringomyelia was extensive.

Detailed histology of the neural plaque (using myelin stains) shows that there is a gross disorganisation of the white matter, so that the long tracts are not recognisable, but short internuncial tracts clearly exist. Although the grey matter is not fully organised into ventral and dorsal horns, there is a clear relationship of neurone clusters to the ventral nerve roots. These histological studies of the plaque indicate that the disorganised development precludes afferent and efferent long tracts developing between the plaque and the normal spinal segments, and there is clearly the likelihood of an upper motor neurone lesion from the uppermost segment involved in the plaque downwards.

When the spinal cord above the myeloschisis is studied with myelin stains, the posterior columns are strikingly narrowed, which again reflects the failure of development of these long conducting tracts throughout the plaque. There is considerable degeneration of the ependyma and grey matter on the surface of the myeloschitic plaques prior to birth, and this degeneration continues, particularly if the plaque is not surgically covered within the first few hours of life.

Developmental Pathology of the Cerebral Lesions

Less attention has been paid to the embryogenesis of the cranial lesions associated with spina bifida than to the spinal ones. In a full description of a 95mm (16 week) human spina bifida fetus, the major features of the tectal and hindbrain malformations are recorded, as well as the encephalocranial disproportion manifested in the posterior fossa, the accompanying slight dilatation of the lateral ventricles, and the shortening and widening of the aqueduct of Sylvius (Brocklehurst 1969*a*, see Fig. 1.6). In the studies of rat fetuses with spina bifida after Trypan blue treatment, similar midbrain and hindbrain abnormalities associated with encephalocranial disproportion are described near term (Warkany 1971, see Fig. 1.7). The same author observed that in some of the malformed fetuses aqueduct stenosis accompanied by hydrocephalus was the only malformation, and that the stenosis preceded the hydrocephalus in these cases. He thought this was an independent phenomenon from the hydrocephalus associated with spina bifida, and that the latter followed upon the obstruction resulting from the brainstem malformation. The development of the lesions of the aqueduct, and the relationship of this to hydrocephalus in spina bifida has already been discussed in Chapter 2.

Pathology of Progressive Hydrocephalus

The hydrocephalic process begins to occur towards the end of intra-uterine development: examination of the ventricles in newborn patients with spina bifida aperta lesions shows dilatation to be present in nearly all cases, although the skull circumference may not be abnormally increased (Lorber 1961). The ventricular dilatation results in rupture of the ependymal lining, extracellular oedema (CSF) in the periventricular white matter, followed by subependymal gliosis and fibre disruption (Weller *et al.* 1969). There is now considerable evidence that in hydrocephalus (if not normally in the human) transventricular absorption of CSF occurs (Brocklehurst 1968*b*, 1972*b*), and these histological and electron microscopic appearances are compatible with this process. Granholm (1968) showed that the total water content of the hydrocephalic brain was no greater than normal, and the assumption is that the subependymal oedema must be entirely a local phenomenon.

Dilatation of the lateral ventricles is accompanied by thinning of the cortex: this is more pronounced at the vertex, and at the occipital and frontal poles (Emery and Svitok 1968). There is dilatation of the third ventricle, considerable thinning of the corpus callosum, and dilatation of the suprapineal recess. These dilatations result in stretching of the components of the limbic lobe (around the corpus callosum) and also in stretching of the long fronto-parietal association fibres in the centrum semi-ovale of the hemispheres.

The enlargement of the cranial vault, which follows the ventricular dilatation and raised intracranial pressure, is accompanied by enlargement of the fontanelles and stretching of the thin membranes which constitute the cranial sutures. Distension and protrusion of the frontal bones is particularly striking (the so-called 'frontal bossing'), and this results in some flattening of the orbital roof.

With the passage of time the hydrocephalic process tends to undergo spontaneous arrest, and although the nature of this still remains to be completely defined, it can be assumed that the dilatation itself, and the development of transventricular absorption (and possibly spontaneous ventriculostomy) offsets the increased pressure, and dilatation ceases.

Developmental Pathology of Foot Deformities

The varieties of club foot so commonly associated with spina bifida, *e.g.* congenital talipes equino-varus, talipes calcaneo-valgus, and the 'rocker-bottom' foot deformity, are basically due to the unopposed action of muscle groups around the ankle joint and intrinsic joints of the foot (Sharrard 1962). The various deformities can be correlated with the absent myotomes and the diminished size of the peripheral nerves which are the secondary results of the lower motor neurone lesions at the level of the plaque. There is another group of foot deformities associated with total paraplegia due to upper motor neurone lesions, and these deformities appear to be positional and result from intra-uterine pressure on paraplegic limbs that are pressed against the trunk (Lendon and Ráliš 1971, Ráliš 1974). (See Chapter 9.)

Developmental Pathology of Deformities of the Spinal Column

In describing and studying the congenital lumbar kyphosis which is so commonly

37

associated with a thoraco-lumbar or high lumbar spina bifida lesion, Barson (1965) has correlated the fixed position of the neural plaque with suppression of the development of the underlying mesodermal somites which give rise to the vertebral column. Thus, at the level of the lesion, the ventral aspects of the vertebrae do not lengthen, and the dorsal aspects lengthen into a keel consisting of the fused derivatives of the everted pedicles. In this way, a striking congenital kyphosis is produced.

In a similar fashion, the vertebrae underlying the asymmetrical hemimyeloschisis lesion ('hemi-myelocele') are retarded in unilateral growth, and this becomes the concavity of a fixed primary scoliosis (the convexity being the side with the more normal cord).

Another primary mesodermal abnormality giving rise to spinal deformity is the occurrence of hemivertebrae or 'butterfly' vertebrae, which may be sited well on the cephalic side of the spina bifida aperta lesion.

Post-natal Development

Postural stresses add to the lower limb and spinal deformities throughout later infancy and childhood (see Chapter 9 on orthopaedic management).

There is a small and quite interesting group of patients who develop very unstable spines, which may go into extremes of lordosis or alternating scoliosis. This appears to be associated with severe hydrocephalus, mental retardation, and a lumbo-sacral myelomeningocele lesion. The upper limbs show hypotonicity and tremor, and the infants often show nystagmus and dysarthria. It seems likely that this deformity is a progressive neurological deficit secondary to hydromyelia of the cervical spinal cord which develops into a syringomyelia, plus the severe cerebellar component of the brainstem abnormality (Brocklehurst, *unpublished observations*).

The neural plaque itself undergoes progressive degeneration throughout infancy and childhood (whether it is covered with skin or not), and this increases the proportion of lower motor neurone lesions in the spina bifida syndrome.

In a similar fashion, the bladder with upper or lower motor lesions disturbing its detrusor function and sphincter activity may be spastic or flaccid at birth, and undergoes progressive dilatation. Subsequent hydronephrosis and renal failure will then occur (see Chapter 11).

Lesions Secondary to Surgical Procedures

Early closure of spina bifida aperta lesions prevents infection of the neural plaque and spinal cord. It is less common to find acute purulent meningitis occurring nowadays. However, chronic meningitis with granular ependymitis, arachnoiditis and meningeal vasculitis are by no means rare, particularly with recurrent shunt infections.

The insertion of ventriculo-atrial or ventriculo-peritoneal shunts has introduced a whole group of secondary lesions. The ventricles of the brain rapidly return to a more or less normal size following a successful shunting procedure, but this process quite often results in brain or choroid plexus impinging upon the tip of the ventricular catheter, which then becomes occluded and hydrocephalus recurs. Repeated passage of a ventricular catheter through the cortex, or the repeated needling of the cortex to reach the ventricles can produce diverticula which are like porencephalic cysts, since they extend from the ventricular wall outwards towards the cortical surface.

The distal end of the shunt placed in the atrium of the heart may give rise to recurrent emboli which land in the pulmonary vascular tree and produce secondary pulmonary hypertension (Erdohazi et *al*. 1966), or thrombosis around the catheter tip may occur and block the superior vena cava. Chronic infection of a ventriculo-atrial shunt results in septicaemia with hepatosplenamegaly and anaemia.

Successful shunting of the severely hydrocephalic infant results not only in a collapse of the cerebral ventricles towards the normal size but a reduction in the whole cranial vault. The previously stretched membraneous bone at the site of the sutures undergoes ossification abnormally quickly, and premature fusion of the sutures results in craniosynostosis.

The cardiac catheters in ventriculo-atrial shunts can become detached and curled up in the heart or in the pulmonary arteries, or they may be lost down the inferior vena cava. Ventriculo-peritoneal shunts can give rise to peritonitis and intestinal obstruction.

CHAPTER 4

Relationship of Pathological Lesions to Clinical Manifestations

Spinal Lesion and Lower Limb Function

Clinical examination of surviving older children and adults with spina bifida lesions commonly reveals a paraplegia of lower motor neurone type associated with wasting and flaccidity, and the tradition arose that this was the basic pathological lesion in the spinal cord. The increased experience of examining neonatal infants with spina bifida lesions (using the type of clinical neurological assessment outlined in Chapter 6) has demonstrated the following varieties of lesion:—

1. A complete spastic paraplegia

The lower limbs do not move when the child is awake, alert, and moving the upper limbs vigorously. A sensory level can be determined above which the child responds to pinprick in a general fashion by moving the arms and crying. Below this level, the response to pinprick or cutaneous stimulation is a segmental or inter-segmental reflex consisting of flexion or adduction movements of the ipsilateral or contralateral limb, and the muscles are well developed and have increased tone. Manipulation of the lower limbs will also produce movement in response to stretching of the muscles. This is basically an upper motor neurone lesion and the sensory and motor level is at the spinal cord segment which is uppermost in the neural plaque accompanying the spina bifida lesion. The pathology is a myeloschisis accompanying a thoraco-lumbar spina bifida.

2. A complete flaccid paraplegia

A few, some, or all of the lower limb movements are absent when the child is awake, crying, and moving the upper limbs, and the corresponding dermatomes (see Chapter 6) are analgesic to pinprick. The paralysed muscles do not respond to cutaneous stimulation, they are noticeably wasted, and on handling they are hypotonic and no movements are produced in response to stretch. The sensory/motor level corresponds to the spinal segment which is uppermost in the neural plaque, and this is basically a lower motor neurone lesion. The pathology is a myelomeningocele, containing either a terminal myeloschisis involving the conus medullaris, or segments of myelodysplasia. A flaccid paraplegia at birth may also be produced by the effect of birth trauma on an exposed neural plaque, converting what would have been, in the case of a frank myeloschisis, an upper motor neurone lesion into a lower motor neurone lesion, the sensory and motor level of the paraplegia being sometimes a little higher than might be expected from the anatomical level of the myeloschisis. This suggests that the birth trauma affects the spinal cord as it comes out of the spinal canal to become involved in the spina bifida lesion (Stark and Drummond 1971).

3. A complete mixed paraplegia

Immediately below the general sensory level the limbs are flaccid and hypalgesic, but distal to this, movements consisting of limited segmental and intersegmental reflexes can be elicited by direct stimulation. The infant is not aroused to general activity anywhere below the main sensory level. This is a mixed upper and lower motor neurone lesion, and the pathology is a myeloschisis or myelodysplasia, usually with some degree of accompanying myelomeningocele.

4. An incomplete flaccid paraplegia

This is similar to 3, but stimulation of the distal segments in which movements occur also arouses the child generally, the intervening segments being flaccid and paralysed. This is an incomplete lesion of lower motor neurone type, and the pathology is usually a myelomeningocele in the mid-to-lower lumbar region with an accompanying myelodysplasia.

5. A spastic paraparesis

This is a rare group in which there is apparent upper motor neurone control of all segments down to the lower sacral ones, and preservation of sensation which arouses the child, but the limbs are paretic with spasticity on handling. This is a partial upper motor neurone lesion affecting the pyramidal tracts, and the pathology is a myelodysplasia associated with minimal spina bifida aperta, or, a myelodysplasia, with or without diastematomyelia, associated with a spina bifida occulta.

6. A monoplegia

This is the asymmetrical lesion in which the lower limb on the side of the convexity of the lumbar scoliosis has apparently normal motor function and tone, and the limb on the concave side is spastic with reflex activity and is subject to an upper motor neurone lesion. The sensory findings are variable and not necessarily crossed, and the pathology is the hemi-myelocele (see Chapter 3), which is really a unilateral myeloschisis or myelodysplasia.

7. Normal

The lower limbs show normal motor power and tone, and full response to pinprick. The spina bifida lesion is a meningocele, a minimal myelomeningocele with the sac containing a few neural filaments, or one of the rarer cervical or upper thoracic saccular lesions containing a diverticulum from the central canal surrounded by glial tissue, which has been termed the 'true myelocele' (see Chapter 3).

Spinal reflex activity in spina bifida patients was noted by Guthkelch (1964) and by Brocklehurst et al. (1967a, b, opera cit.). In the same year, Stark and Baker described the upper and lower motor neurone lesions found by clinical neurological examination of neonates with spina bifida, and related them to the pathology of the spinal cord lesions. They found evidence of function in an isolated distal portion of the cord in 50 per cent of their patients studied, and in 20 per cent the reflex function was extensive. 43.4 per cent of their material showed the pattern described in Type 2 (page 56). In 1971, Stark and Drummond published the results of another study in which the same kind of clinical neurological assessment was supplemented by electro-myographic recordings and stimulation of the neural plaque. They confirmed that muscles derived from segments progressively caudal in the spinal cord were more likely to show an upper motor neurone lesion and spinal reflex activity. Furthermore, they showed, by plaque stimulation combined with EMG, that there was some degree of lower motor neurone innervation to the majority of muscles in the lower limbs of these infants, and a striking absence of denervation patterns. However, quite a large percentage of these apparently innervated muscles showed no clinical activity, *i.e.* by electromyographic criteria the majority of the muscles should have shown upper motor neurone lesions, but clinical examination, even in the warm newborn infant with spina bifida aperta, will frequently show an apparent lower motor neurone type of paraplegia. The studies by Brocklehurst *et al.* (1967*a, b*) on infants undergoing early closure of spina bifida aperta lesions confirmed the low threshold for excitability of the neural plaque, and how, in the asymmetrical lesion, the dysplastic side is more easily stimulated than the normal one. In the awake newborn infant, touching the open myeloschisis will often produce bilateral withdrawal reflexes in the lower limbs, and, when the infant is lying supine during the clinical examination, similar movements will be produced by auto-stimulation (see Chapter 6).

These findings correlate well with the neuropathology of the spinal lesions, for both in the frank myeloschisis and in the myelodysplasia, anterior horn cells are abundantly present in the affected segments throughout later fetal development and at the time of birth (see Chapter 3). In the neonatal period, many of these segmental lower motor neurones are active and have internuncial connections, and the anatomical basis for spinal reflex movements is clearly present. In these circumstances, the level of the upper motor neurone lesion is basically determined by the point at which the myeloschisis or dysplasia interferes with development and myelination of cortico-spinal tracts. To this basic lesion may be added the effect of mechanical distortion of the junction between neural plaque and spinal cord by birth trauma, or by the progressive accumulation of fluid which distends the sac of a myelomeningo-cele, both causing superimposed lower motor neurone lesions. Furthermore, the surface degeneration of the neural plaque (which has already begun to occur during later fetal development) is increased by exposure, drying and infection after birth. Frank infection of the spina bifida aperta lesion with ascending meningitis produces a rapidly progressive flaccid paraplegia and is often fatal. Spontaneous epithelialisation of the untreated plaque is also accompanied by degeneration, and the lower motor neurone picture supervenes. It is interesting that closure of the open spina bifida lesion within a few hours of birth appears to preserve the lower motor neurone function, and the clinical manifestations of the upper motor neurone type of spastic paraplegia will persist for weeks or months. However, even in these cases, the lesion ultimately becomes a basically flaccid paraplegia.

In the Type 1 lesions, the appearance of the lower limbs in the newborn infant is often normal, but sometimes there is a type of symmetrical talipes equinovarus deformity. This appears to be the result of the flexed spastic limbs being compressed against the trunk during later fetal development (Ráliš 1974, see Chapter 3). Later in life, these children develop very characteristic postures of their lower limbs, with abduction of the hips and spastic plantar flexion of the toes, which is similar to the deformity seen in an adult with a spastic hemiplegia (see Chapter 9).

Infants with the Type 2 lesions characteristically show the deformities of muscle imbalance described by Sharrard (1962): genu recurvatum from the unopposed action of the lumbar spinal segments 3 and 4; calcaneal deformities of the ankle from unopposed lumbar 4/5 segments; talipes equinovarus deformities from unopposed lumbar 5/sacral 1; and 'rocker-bottom' foot deformities from intrinsic muscle failure at S1, S2 level (see Chapter 9).

Infants with the Type 3 and Type 4 lesions show muscle imbalance less frequently and the lower limbs are not so characteristically deformed.

In the Type 5 lesion, particularly when the spastic paraparesis results from a myelodysplasia with diastematomyelia and a spina bifida occulta lesion, there is often a limited lower motor neurone lesion or root lesion affecting L5 or S1, and giving rise to a unilateral talipes deformity; this has been termed the 'orthopaedic syndrome' (James and Lassman 1960). The spastic paraparesis may gradually progress in the diastematomyelia patients, and even the unilateral lower motor neurone lesion may become more obvious in later childhood. This phenomenon is more likely to be due to repeated trauma around the diastematomyelia spur than to any other mechanism (Guthkelch 1974).

The monoplegia associated with the Type 6 lesion is characteristically spastic, with plantar flexion of the ankle.

Spinal Lesion and Vertebral Column Function

The primary deformities of the vertebral column and their developmental pathology have been discussed in Chapter 3. Secondary increase in lumbar kyphosis occurring in later childhood has been related to the weight of the trunk in the upright child and the unopposed pull of muscles such as the psoas and quadratus lumborum, which have innervation from upper lumbar segments and are stretched across the cavity of the lumbar kyphosis to reach their insertion (Drennan 1970).

Increase in lateral deformities may result from progressive development of a lower motor neurone degeneration in segments controlling the small intraspinal muscles, as in anterior poliomyelitis.

Spinal Lesion and Bladder Function

Bladder innervation is from the second, third and fourth sacral segments, and since nearly all spina bifida aperta lesions have structural abnormalities of the cord at or above this level, there will be neurological abnormalities affecting the bladder in well over 90 per cent. In many cases the lesion is of upper motor neurone type, and the automatic bladder function hardly distinguishable from that of a normal neonate, although manometric studies and urological investigations may show that the bladder is in fact spastic within the first few days of birth, and the sphincter tone is abnormally increased.

Spina bifida lesions which affect primarily the sacrum are associated with a lower motor neurone lesion in the tip of the conus medullaris, and the bladder is flaccid from the outset, easily distended, and shows dribbling incontinence in the neonatal

43

period. In these infants the flaccidity of the levator ani and anal sphincters is also obvious on clinical examination (see Chapter 6). Again, the EMG studies indicate that the segments have, nevertheless, a lower motor neurone supply in the majority of cases, and there is occasionally some clinical recovery of this lower motor neurone function. Mixed patterns have also been obtained in manometric studies, and Stark (1968) has again related these findings to the neuropathology of the cord lesions. In later infancy and childhood the bladder tends to become atonic with outflow obstruction, whether it was initially flaccid or spastic. The failure of successful evacuation leads to the secondary changes so common in the urinary tracts of these infants (see Chapter 11).

Brainstem Malformation and Respiratory and Bulbar Function

The frequency with which infants with spina bifida lesions and hydrocephalus demonstrate bouts of apnoea and stridor is well known to clinicians, but the cause of these has only been recently elucidated. Bilateral abductor paralysis of the vocal cords secondary to the brainstem malformation in spina bifida has been described (Snow 1965), and this is undoubtedly one factor. Progressive hydrocephalus is another factor, and is acting by compression and displacement of the malformed medulla. Relief of the hydrocephalus in the neonatal period will often favourably affect both the bouts of apnoea and the respiratory stridor. Wealthall (1974), by monitoring the respiratory patterns and blood gases of these infants, has shown that there is a basic abnormality which persists even after a tracheostomy and relief of the hydrocephalus; throughout the first few weeks of life the level of the capillary pCO_2 progressively rises, and the infants develop true periodic respiration, with bradycardia when they go to sleep (sleep apnoea). The whole syndrome is thought to be a combination of upper airway obstruction with the primary malformation of the medulla, which results in some dissociation across the cervical medullary junction similar to that seen in adults with sleep apnoea following bilateral high cervical percutaneous cordotomy (the so-called 'Ondine's curse'). This disturbance in respiratory control is considered to be a cause of sudden, unexplained death in spina bifida infants between nine and 12 weeks, and it is also recorded that these infants will often show spontaneous recovery after the 12-week stage.

Clinical manifestations of hydrocephalus

The pathology of the progressive hydrocephalus which leads to ventricular dilatation was described in Chapter 3. In many infants with spina bifida aperta lesions, this process is already present at birth, and in a minority the secondary enlargement of the skull circumference is also present at that time. In the majority, the hydrocephalus, if untreated, causes progressive skull circumference expansion in the neonatal period, and if there is a meningocele sac associated with the spina bifida lesion this will often become progressively distended. The fontanelles become tense and bulging, and compression of the sac will increase this tension. In addition to the brainstem disturbances described above, the infants will often show a downcasting of the eyes, with an increased exposure of the sclera as the hydrocephalus progresses. This downcasting can be rapidly relieved by treating the hydrocephalus and has been related to dilatation of the suprapineal recess causing a 'tectal plate syndrome' and depressing upward gaze (as in the well recognised syndrome of a pineal tumour).

The increase of intracranial tension from the progressive hydrocephalus ultimately compresses the cerebral veins and increases the sagittal sinus venous pressure (Norrell *et al.* 1969). This causes dilatation of the emissary veins, and these have been observed in post-mortem examinations of these infants (Blaauw 1970). Clinically, the infant shows dilated veins in the frontal and parietal regions which immediately collapse on relief of the hydrocephalus. In the untreated case, progressive enlargement can occur until the skull is huge, and may contain over a litre of cerebrospinal fluid (see Fig. 8.1). In addition to the respiratory manifestations described above, there is a general irritability of the child and hypertonicity of the limbs as the hydrocephalus progresses.

Arrested Hydrocephalus

Surgical arrest of hydrocephalus stops the abnormal skull expansion, and the vault becomes firm and may ossify abnormally early. In these circumstances, recurrence of the hydrocephalus (from a blocked ventriculo-atrial shunt) is accompanied by rapid clinical deterioration, with a very high pressure, lowered level of consciousness, and apnoea.

Spontaneous arrest of hydrocephalus, which probably occurs by increased transventricular absorption of CSF combined with the reduction of pulse pressure by the enlarged ventricular volume, is quite common by the age of five years, and the child then maintains normal skull circumference growth.

There is a small but important group of infants with low lumbo-sacral or sacral myelomeningocele lesions, a normal skull circumference at birth, and no obvious cranial dysplasia. In these infants, the hydrocephalus occurs without much ventricular enlargement and there is strikingly raised intracranial pressure so that apnoea can rapidly supervene, and this well before there is significant increase in the skull circumference.

Mental Function and Personality Changes in Hydrocephalus

In 1962, Ingram and Naughton pointed out that among their children with so-called 'cerebral palsy', there was a group with varying mixtures of cerebral diplegia and ataxia, who, judged by their skull circumference and previous history, appeared to have hydrocephalus and that the psychological testing in this group confirmed the clinical impression that the verbal I.Q. was much higher than the performance I.Q. One qualitative aspect of this is the personality of the child who is sociable, loves to chatter a great deal, and appears to be bright, but it becomes rapidly clear that there is no depth to the knowledge, nor any persistence in concentrating on a subject or task; this was given the term 'cocktail party syndrome' by Hadenius *et al.* (1962). Parsons (1968) could not correlate this apparent verbal facility of hydrocephalic children with any particular facility for learning words or misusing them when allowance was made for the lower I.Q.s of the group studied, but Fleming (1968) did show a significantly greater amount of inappropriate verbal responses in these children, in addition to their apparent verbosity. In a more recent study, Miller and

45

Sethi (1971) showed that the hydrocephalic children had quantitative deficiencies in the perception of visuo-spatial relationships.

The dilatation of the cerebral ventricles in hydrocephalus occurs at the expense of the long association fibres from frontal to parietal regions (which run in the centrum semi-ovale of the cerebral hemispheres), increased stretching and thinning of the corpus callosum, and the circumventing fibres of the hippocampal gyrus and fornices (which constitute part of the postulated 'limbic lobe'). It is conceivable that the pressure atrophy of these structures is in some way responsible for the particular personality features, although it might be expected that the limbic lobe lesions would be manifested more in terms of short-term memory loss. There must be some critical level at which these lesions secondary to ventricular dilatation become clinically manifest, for it is well known that many patients with confirmed hydrocephalus and some degree of ventricular dilatation are able to achieve quite normal mental function and a high I.Q.

CHAPTER 5

The Epidemiology of Spina Bifida

Incidence and Regional Variations

Figures for the incidence of spina bifida have now been collected from a number of centres in different countries, and are usually given in terms of the number per 1,000 total births. In these epidemiological studies a very close relationship has been observed between the incidence of spina bifida and anencephaly, and a less close relationship between spina bifida and congenital hydrocephalus.

The natural incidence of spina bifida varies considerably in different parts of the world: Table 5.I (Laurence 1969) shows a range from 0.3 per 1,000 births in Japan to over four per 1,000 births in some parts of the British Isles. Studies from America show an incidence in general lower than in Europe, with important ethnic variations (see below), and Hewitt (1963) found that the mortality attributed to spina bifida was two to three times greater on the Atlantic than on the Pacific coast, both in Canada and in the United States. Figures from Israel show an incidence of 1.05 per 1,000 in 1958, dropping to 0.44 per 1,000 in 1968 (Naggan 1971).

Earlier studies from the British Isles showed important regional variations; the high incidence in South Wales and Dublin (4.1 and 4.2 per 1,000 total births respectively) contrasted with the low incidence in East Anglia and Birmingham (1.6 per 1,000 total births) (Record and McKeown 1949, Brocklehurst 1968a, Laurence 1966).

Even more detailed population studies have been made for the South Wales area and, taking neural tube malformations as a whole, the incidence in the valleys of east and west Glamorgan and Monmouth was strikingly higher than in the rest of these two counties (Richards et al. 1972). In these population studies in Wales, no correlation was found between the area differences and other demographic features such as social class, parity, maternal age, ethnic composition, and population movements between the regions. Naggan and MacMahon (1967) studied the immigration effect upon the incidence of spina bifida in Boston and found that it was relatively higher among the Boston-Irish and those with half Irish marriages, but still the incidence in ex-Irish families was less high than in Belfast.

The stillbirth rate for spina bifida infants is about 25 per cent and this reduces the number per 1,000 live births to a range of from three to 1.6; commonly given average is two per 1,000 live births (Record and McKeown 1949; Doran and Guthkelch 1961; Swinyard and Shahani 1966; Laurence 1966, Laurence et al. 1968a, 1968b; Laurence 1969).

Seasonal Variation

In 1962, Guthkelch pointed out that analysis of the incidence of spina bifida could be related to the month of birth of the infants. Both the Scottish and Manchester series

TABLE 5.1

Incidence of neural tube malformations in various centres

Centre / Incidence per 1,000 births	South Wales (Laurence et al. 1968a and b)	Liverpool (Smithells 1967)	Belfast (Stevenson and Warnock 1959)	Southampton (Williamson 1965)	Birmingham (McKeown and Record 1960)	Charleston (Alter 1962) White	Charleston (Alter 1962) Negro	Alexandria* (Stevenson et al. 1966)	Japan (Neel 1958)
Anencephaly	3.5	3.1	4.6	1.9	2.0	1.2	0.2	3.6	0.6
Spina Bifida	4.1	3.7	2.2	3.2	2.8	1.5	0.6	2.0	0.3
Hydrocephalus	0.5	0.5	1.5	0.9	1.8	0.8	1.1	2.0	0.3
Total	8.1	7.3	8.3	6.0	6.6	3.5	1.9	7.6	1.2

*Not a population study

TABLE 5.II

Estimated recurrence risks for spina bifida or anencephaly or both (from Smith 1972)

Family History	Estimated risk
One sib affected	5.5
Parent and sib affected/two sibs affected	13.0
Three sibs affected	20.6
One sib and a second-degree relative affected	9.2
One sib and a third-degree relative affected	7.3
One sib affected, no other family history	3.7

showed that the number born per month between December and May was on the average higher than those born between June and November. The inference that spring and summer conceptions had a greater liability to develop spina bifida has been confirmed by others, and Carter (1974) has pointed out that the situation is reversed in the southern hemisphere, which suggests a relationship between the occurrence of spina bifida and the length of daytime.

Racial Differences

A number of studies have shown that while the incidence of spina bifida (and anencephaly) is high in Europe and particularly in Ireland, it is low in Negro and Mongolian races (see Table 5.I). The races with a high incidence tend to take the high incidence with them when migrating (see figures of the Boston survey above). Racial differences in the occurrence of other central nervous system malformations are well known, and anterior cranial meningocele and encephalocele is much commoner amongst Mongolian and Chinese races.

Many surveys have shown that the higher social classes (1 and 2) have a lower incidence of spina bifida and anencephaly, and this was confirmed in a survey of the incidence of these conditions among Jews in Israel (Naggan 1971). However, when looking at the incidence among Jews in Boston, Naggan and MacMahon (1967) did not find any increase at the lower ends of the social scale.

Environmental Factors

The effect of migration upon ethnic differences in the occurrence of spina bifida and anencephaly suggests that there are also environmental factors involved. In 1972, Renwick put forward the hypothesis that the environmental factor could be an unidentified substance present in certain potato tubers, a hypothesis based upon the epidemiological data and the history of the potato crops in the British Isles. The correlations put forward by Renwick have not been widely substantiated, but one or two other studies have also related the incidence of this condition to dietary factors such as canned meats and tea drinking (*see* Carter 1974).

Genetic Factors

In any large series of spina bifida cases, a positive family history is obtained in around 10 per cent, and many special studies have been made of these families (Smithells *et al.* 1968, Laurence 1969). In these studies, the incidence of anencephaly and spina bifida occurring in the siblings and relatives of index cases are usually studied together. The chance of neural tube defects in siblings born after a spina bifida or anencephaly case is just over five per cent and the second malformation is more likely to be of the same sort as the first than different. After two malformed infants the chances of having another are between 10 and 15 per cent. With a knowledge of the family history, the risk of a recurrence of spina bifida or anencephaly can be estimated from these figures and given to the parents either from such a table as 5.II, or by using a computer programme (Smith 1972). This is of importance in relationship to genetic counselling (see Chapter 11).

There is a slight preponderance of females over males of about 1.3 to 1.0 in most spina bifida series. The concurrence of spina bifida in monozygotic co-twins is about 20 per cent and in dizygotic six per cent.

The nature of the genetic pattern revealed by these studies has been described as a polygenically inherited predisposition (Laurence 1969, *opus cit.*), and with the other epidemiological features, these studies provide important evidence that spina bifida and anencephaly are associated conditions with a multifactorial aetiology (Carter 1974, *opus cit.*).

CHAPTER 6

Assessment and Management of Infants with Obvious Spinal Lesion

Initial Referral and Travel

Spina bifida aperta lesions are usually noticed immediately after birth. Infants with this condition should receive expert assessment and management within the first few hours of life. In many cases this means referral to a centre within an area or region where there is both the neurological and paediatric expertise required for this kind of assessment, and the surgical facilities for early operative treatment if this is the course advisable. The open spinal lesion should be covered with saline-soaked gauze, and the infant transported in an incubator to maintain body heat. It is preferable that the general nature of the condition and the possibility of surgical treatment be discussed with the mother before transferral, and that the father accompany the child. The obstetrical notes and a sample of the mother's blood should be sent with the child, and the unit to which the infant is referred should be warned of the child's arrival.

History Taking

The history is brief and should be taken from the obstetrical notes and the parent available; any family history of congenital malformations of the nervous system is important, and the details of the pregnancy, labour and delivery should be recorded. Obstetrical abnormalities and complications of labour are relatively frequent in this condition.

Clinical Examination of Spina Bifida Patients

The newborn infant with a spina bifida lesion is initially assessed for general health and robustness; the height and weight are recorded and the examination of the cardiovascular, respiratory and alimentary system performed, particularly with a view to elucidating any other major congenital abnormalities.

The neurological examination consists firstly of inspection, palpation of the skull, measurement of the skull circumference, and recording of the size and tensions of the anterior, posterior and lateral fontanelles, if present. The configuration of the skull and the shape of the posterior fossa are also recorded. When the skull circumference is already abnormally increased at birth then hydrocephalus is regarded as clinically established (see Chapter 8).

Transillumination of the skull in a dark room is not a customary part of this initial examination, but it should be performed if the skull is particularly enlarged, the anterior fontanelle particularly tense, or there is any suggestion from palpation and percussion that there may be an asymmetrical collection of fluid within the cranial vault. When the examination is properly performed, fluid-containing cavities within the cranial vault will illuminate brightly: the test is positive when there is extreme hydrocephalus or the condition called hydranencephaly, or where there is an asymmetrical large collection of fluid associated with porencephaly, or diencephalic cysts.

The absence or presence of the suck, startle and grasp reflexes, and the vigour of the cry and the respiratory pattern give a good indication of the basic neurological activity of the infant. External ocular movements with neck rotation, pupillary responses to light, and examination of the fundi are performed. Facial sensation and facial muscle power in response to pinprick are recorded, and the tongue, palatal and pharyngeal muscle power assessed in gagging, crying and swallowing. The sterno-mastoid and trapezius muscles are assessed for bulk, power, and any evidence of birth injury. Inspection of the neck and shoulders may show congenital abnormalities of the cervical spine which are sometimes present in spina bifida patients. Neck rotation may be used to elicit tonic neck reflexes in order to assess continuity of the cortico-spinal tract to the upper and lower limbs. The upper limbs are inspected and palpated for power and tone.

The lesion on the back is measured for its maximal diameter; its site in relationship to the lowest ribs, lumbar spine, sacro-iliac joint or iliac crest is accurately recorded and listed as thoraco-lumbar, lumbo-sacral, lumbar, sacral, cervical or thoracic. The accurate anatomical determination of the lesion gives a good indication of the likely segmental level of the neurological deficit (see Chapter 4).

The nature of the covering of the lesion is recorded as being either membraneous, abnormal skin, or normal skin, and a note made as to whether the sac is leaking or intact. The presence or absence of visible neural tissue in the midline, or raw granulation tissue which may lie over the neural plaque, is also recorded.

The examination of the lower limbs is approached carefully; if the infant is lying quietly then the neurological pin is run lightly from the sacral region down the back and then up the front of the legs until a level is reached at which the whole infant is aroused to a general response. Local movements of the lower limbs in response to pinprick may occur well below the segmental level of the spinal lesion and be due to spinal reflexes occurring through the neural plaque (see Chapter 4). If, at this point in the examination, the infant is awake and crying and moving the upper limbs spon-taneously, then the lower limbs are inspected without palpation, and the spontaneous movements analysed in terms of flexion and extension of the hip joint, knee joint, ankle joint and toes respectively. These movements are the true spontaneous movements of the infants' lower limbs and are dependent upon an intact cortico-spinal tract. A particularly sensitive, exposed neural plaque may be stimulated to produce some of these movements by the general mobility of the trunk of the awake infant causing pressure of the neural plaque against the surface on which the infant is lying; this auto-stimulation can be eliminated by turning the awake infant on to his side.

The dermatome areas of the lower limbs and also the myotome values for the various joint movements should be known (see Figs. 6.1 and 6.2). It will usually be found that the true sensory level at which the whole infant arouses to pinprick stimulation will agree mostly with the myotome level to which upper motor neurone control persists. Below this level, movements may be elicited by handling or stimulating the feet, thighs or perineum; flexion withdrawal, crossed extension and other movements may also be produced quite easily. These spinal reflex movements do not usually disturb the whole patient and they should be recorded in the examination; they occur more commonly in the infants with the high thoraco-lumbar lesions accompanied by a total myeloschisis, particularly when the plaque is in good condition and the infant is warm (Type 1 paralysis, see Chapter 4 and Fig. 6.5).

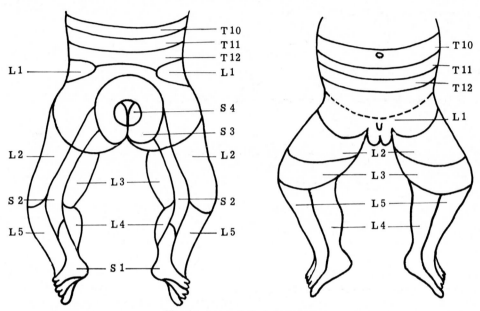

Fig. 6.1. Lower limb dermatomes.

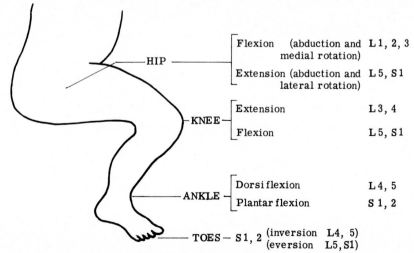

Fig. 6.2. Lower limb myotomes.

53

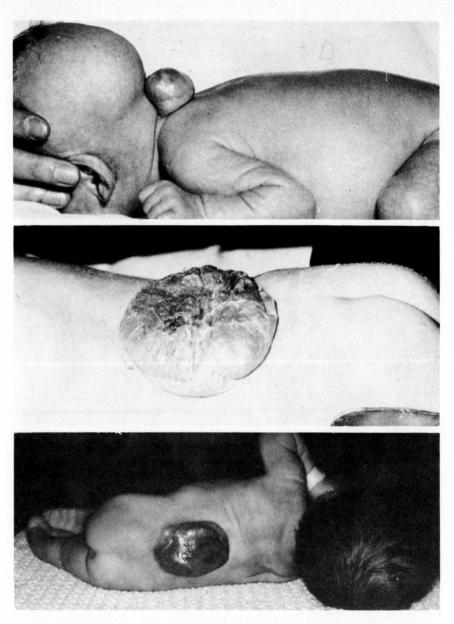

Fig. 6.3 (*top*). Infant with cervical meningocele. This infant has normal neurological function of the lower limbs (Type 7) and has a good prognosis (Group A). (Photograph by courtesy of Mr. A. N. Guthkelch.)

Fig. 6.4 (*middle*). (See also Figs. 9.1, 9.2.) Infant with lumbar myelomeningocele. This infant has a lower motor neurone lesion affecting ankle movement (Type 2) and a moderately good prognosis (Group B).

Fig. 6.5 (*bottom*). Infant with thoraco-lumbar myeloschisis. This infant has an upper motor neurone paralysis of the lower limbs (Type 1) and a poor prognosis (Group C).

54

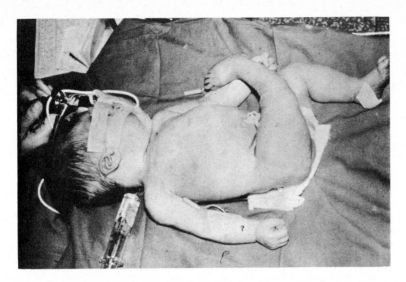

Fig. 6.6. Infant with hemi-myeloschisis. This infant has an asymmetrical lower limb paralysis, or monoplegia (Type 6) and a relatively good prognosis (Group D). (From Duckworth 1968.)

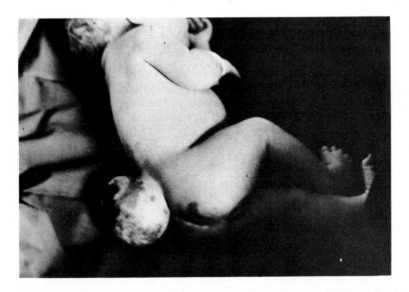

Fig. 6.7. Infant with low sacral myelomeningocele. This infant has a minimal flaccid paralysis affecting ankle plantar flexion (Type 2) and a good prognosis (Group B). Rarely, this type of lesion is associated with normal lower limb function (Type 7) and a very good prognosis (Group A). (See also Figs. 9.3, 9.4, 9.5.) (Photograph by courtesy of Dr. Richard Pugh.)

In the lumbar and sacral lesions, the lower limbs will show a lower motor neurone type of lesion to a greater or lesser extent (see Figs. 6.4, 6.7, 9.1 to 9.5 and Chapter 9). When this lower motor neurone lesion appears to be complete (Type 2) in a large number of segments at birth there may be some recovery and the display of spinal reflex movement later, particularly with warming and surgical closure of the lesion.

In the Type 3 paralysis, segments just distal to the rostral end of the spina bifida aperta show flaccidity and a lower motor neurone paralysis; but distal to this, spinal reflexes and spasticity are abundantly present. In the dermatomes of the segments which demonstrate spinal reflex activity, direct stimulation does not produce a general arousal of the infant; the assumption is that the cord pathology is a total myeloschisis with complete loss of long tract continuity, and segmental loss of anterior horn cells (see Chapter 9 and Fig 9.6).

Type 4 is an important variety of this lesion (Type 3), in which stimulation distal to the segments of lower motor neurone paralysis produces not only muscle activity but a striking general arousal of the child so that an incomplete cord lesion must be diagnosed. The exact distribution of lower motor neurone lesions in this case (and these may be actual peripheral nerve lesions) may require time to elucidate, and the amount of cortico-spinal control over the distal spinal cord segments may also take time to demonstrate. Such children, however, may well have important control of the S2, 3 and 4 segments and develop continence.

The Type 5 lesion consists of a spastic paresis from the site of the spina bifida lesion downwards, the spina bifida lesion itself often being relatively superficial and an incomplete myeloschisis or myelodysplasia. In these infants it is clear from the beginning that there is pinprick sensation which produces general arousal right down to the sacral segments and that the lower limb movements, although spastic, are indeed spontaneous. This again is an incomplete spinal lesion and is relatively uncommon.

The Type 6 paralysis is the asymmetrical one in which one lower limb shows good apparent spontaneous muscle activity and general arousal of the infant to pinprick, and the other lower limb has a spastic or flaccid lesion from the level of the spina bifida downwards. The paralysed limb coincides with the concave side of the plaque and the accompanying scoliosis in this hemi-myeloschisis lesion (see Fig. 6.6).

Type 7 is the all too rare situation in which the lower limbs show full spontaneous activity and sensation to pinprick, and the lesion is a low sacral cystic meningocele with no plaque, or the rarer thoracic or cervical meningocele (see Fig. 6.3).

The examination of the lower limbs is not complete without the observation and recording of deformities such as the variety of talipes, genu recurvatum, and congenital dislocation of the hips. Sphincter function may also be estimated; the patulous anus which pouts whenever the child cries, combined with dribbling incontinence, indicates a lower motor neurone lesion of the S2, 3 and 4 segments, and the spastic indrawn anus is accompanied by a bladder with a good micturition stream.

The main features of the neurological examination of these infants has been previously well described (see Guthkelch 1964; Brocklehurst et al. 1967a, 1967b; Stark and Baker 1967; Duckworth and Brown 1970; Stark 1971; Stark and Drummond 1971; and Chapters 9 and 11).

Electrodiagnosis

Although faradic stimulation of the lower limb muscles in newborn infants with spina bifida lesions shows that muscle contraction is present in the majority, it fails to distinguish whether or not the muscle is under normal upper motor neurone control or is under lower motor neurone control only. Muscles which show no faradic response have progressed beyond denervation to wasting and fibrosis.

Electromyographic recording of muscle groups has been a useful research tool; it demonstrates the abundance of lower motor neurone activity which is present in the neonatal period and later. Action potentials, recorded as discharges in bursts while the infant is generally active and moving the arms, are good evidence of lower motor neurone activity which is under upper motor neurone control (*i.e.* normal voluntary movement). Action potentials of abnormal size and duration may be easily elicited by stimulation of the limbs below the level of the spinal lesion, or by direct electrical stimulation of the neural plaque, and the demonstration of lower motor neurone activity which lacks upper motor neurone control is far more extensive when this technique is used. Fibrillation potentials or absence of action potentials indicate lower motor neurone lesions or denervation of the muscle groups being examined. Used in this way, electromyographic studies have shown disappearance of fibrillation potentials and the occurrence of polyphasic potentials, indicating reinnervation after birth and surgical closure (Chantraine *et al.* 1967).

The demonstration of muscle groups with lower motor neurone lesions may be useful in the Type 3 and 4 paralysis defined above, particularly if clinical and electromyographic examination suggests that the segments distal to the level of lower motor neurone lesions have some degree of upper motor neurone control, for the preservation of the affected segments at operation becomes vitally important, and the prognosis for the future correspondingly better informed.

Radiological Investigations (Figs. 6.8, 6.9, 6.10)

Radiographs of the total child in the antero-posterior and lateral positions should be done using large plates and just two exposures. These X-rays will usually include a satisfactory lateral radiograph of the skull, and if not, this should be obtained separately in order to complete the radiological assessment. The total body radiograph in the antero-posterior view shows the level of the spina bifida lesion; this can be identified quite easily by the eversion of the abnormal pedicles and the increased interpedicular distance. The anatomical site of the spina bifida lesion can be clearly demarcated by putting a wire round the spina bifida aperta on the skin prior to the X-ray. Associated mesodermal anomalies such as butterfly or hemivertebrae, double or absent ribs, and gross spinal scoliosis can be identified from these pictures, and such anomalies are more commonly associated with the high thoraco-lumbar lesions with a full myeloschisis (Fig. 6.9). Similarly, the lateral view of the spine will show any associated congenital kyphosis, and occasionally an odd bony projection in association with the spina bifida will be outlined (see Fig. 6.8).

A further advantage of these preliminary total-body radiographs is that they form a basic screening of the heart shape, the lung fields and the gastro-intestinal tract, as well as the position of the hip joints.

The skull radiographs, particularly in the lateral view, may show craniolacunae (see Fig. 6.8), the abnormal size and shape of the foramen magnum and the flattening of the petrous ridges, and the general skull shape. In particular, the depth of the posterior fossa can be assessed quite easily by drawing a line from the external auditory meatus (as it is visualised in the petrous temporal bone) to the internal occipital protruberance (line A-B in Figs. 6.8 and 6.10), and then dropping a perpendicular (line C-D) down to the squamous occipital bone from a point around halfway along A-B. In the normal skull, C-D equals or exceeds half of A-B; in the shallow posterior fossa, C-D is considerably less than half of A-B. A shallow posterior fossa is assocaited with the Cleland-Arnold-Chiari hindbrain malformation, and clinically significant hydrocephalus is almost certain to develop in these cases. Extensive craniolacunae and the other features of cranial dysplasia are associated with severe underlying cerebral dysplasia, hydrocephalus at birth, and likely mental retardation in the future. The radiological features associated with spina bifida which may be shown in plain radiographs are listed in Table 6.I.

TABLE 6.I

Radiographic features associated with severe spina bifida lesions

Spine	Skull
Eversion of pedicles	Craniolacunae
Kyphosis	Shallow posterior fossa
Hemi-vertebrae	Eversion of petrous temporal bones
Double ribs	Enlargement of foramen magnum
Absent ribs	

Factors in Making a Prognosis

The clinical examination (as performed above), combined with the radiographs and perhaps aided by electromyography, will provide a reasonable basis for a prognosis, and in this respect the following classification may be found useful.

Group A

A robust infant with no skull enlargement and a low sacral spina bifida aperta lesion or a limited cystic lesion in the cervical or thoracic region and no neurological deficit detected in the lower limbs or sphincters. The neurological picture is of the Type 7 described previously, and the radiographs will show limited spinal abnormalities and probably a normal skull (Figs. 3.1c 6.3 and 6.10). This infant is likely to walk normally or nearly so, may have normal sphincter control, and is quite likely not to develop hydrocephalus. However, the possibility of not detecting a minimal neurological lower limb or sphincter deficit in the newborn, and the possibility of the development of late hydrocephalus, or the type of early post-operative high pressure hydrocephalus associated with only slightly enlarged ventricles, should provide slight reservations in the prognosis. Untreated, this infant is at risk of losing life or neurological function from infection of the sac and subsequent meningitis.

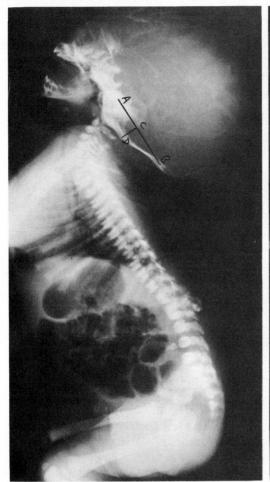

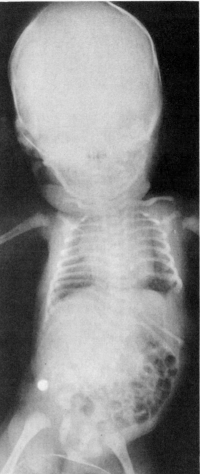

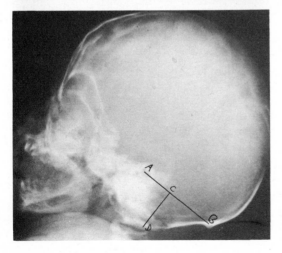

Fig. 6.8 (*above left*). Lateral radiograph of infant with spina bifida showing cranio-lacunae and shallow posterior fossa (see text). These features have a high association with hydrocephalus clinically apparent at birth and future mental retardation.

Fig. 6.9 (*above right*). Antero-posterior radiograph of infant with thoraco-lumbar spina bifida, showing congenital scoliosis and absent ribs.

Fig. 6.10 (*left*). Lateral skull radiograph of spina bifida infant showing no cranio-lacunae and normal posterior fossa (see text).

Group B

A robust infant with an open lumbar or sacral lesion, no skull enlargement at birth, the lower limbs with at least spontaneous hip flexion (L2) and often with knee extension and independent right and left ankle dorsiflexion. Below the level of spontaneous muscle activity there are lower motor neurone lesions affecting intrinsic muscles of the feet, gluteal muscles, perhaps the calf muscles and sometimes the hamstrings and quadriceps. The sphincters may show a lower motor neurone lesion and the feet may have talipes or rocker-bottom deformity. In infants with functioning L3 myotomes, a genu-recurvatum deformity associated with a breech delivery is not uncommon. The back lesion is an obvious myeloschisis or severe myelodysplasia covered with granulation tissue, and it may well be saccular at birth (Figs. 3.1*b*, 6.4, 6.7). The paralysis in these infants is of the Type 2, 3 or 4 described above and the radiographs demonstrate clearly the spinal lesion and show the skull to have a shallow posterior fossa without severe craniolacunae or obvious skull enlargement at this stage. The electromyographic studies in this difficult group may elucidate whether or not the lower limbs have the Type 2, 3, or 4 paralysis (*i.e.* are neurologically complete or incomplete lesions).

Taken as a whole, infants in this group will almost certainly develop hydrocephalus, but successful treatment of this will result in a mental achievement within normal or educable range. Walking will be achieved with considerable orthopaedic help. Incontinence and urinary tract complications secondary to upper or lower motor neurone bladder lesions are inevitable in the majority. Without surgical treatment, further neurological deterioration would occur and the infants would probably die.

Group C

A robust infant with an abnormally increased skull circumference present at birth, an open thoraco-lumbar spina bifida with myeloschisis, no spontaneous lower limb movement, a thoracic general sensory level, and abundant evidence of spinal reflexes (Figs. 3.1*a* and 6.5). The spasticity of the lower limbs is obvious. Sometimes there are accompanying spastic lower limb deformities such as abduction and dislocation of the hips and a spastic talipes equinovarus. The general sensory level coincides with the anatomy of the uppermost segment involved in the obvious myeloschisis, which at birth is usually quite flat. The anus is also spastic and indrawn.

Skull enlargement in this group is obvious, and the fontanelles are of abnormal shape and distended. The shallow posterior fossa can be clinically palpated and confirmed in the lateral skull X-ray. Craniolacunae and the presence of a lumbar kyphus, hemivertebrae and scoliosis, and abnormal rib formations will also be shown. The antero-posterior spinal X-rays show the vertebral features of spina bifida extending from the thoracic to the sacral region. It is noticeable clinically that the sacral segments of the spinal cord (developed from the tail-bud) are covered by normal skin.

The paralysis in this group is of the Type 1 described above; this whole clinical syndrome accounts for almost 50 per cent in any large, unselected series of newborn infants with spina bifida aperta lesions. Electromyography confirms the upper motor neurone lesions and may show various degrees of additional lower motor neurone lesions which will affect sacral segments or sphincters, the lower motor neurone lesions easily progressing or reversing depending upon treatment of the plaque.

Infants in this group will remain totally paraplegic whether they are treated or not, and they are unlikely to be able to use spinal and full lower-limb calipers well enough to achieve a type of pull-through walking. Mental retardation is likely whether the hydrocephalus is treated or not, and incontinence and urinary tract complications are inevitable.

Group D

A robust infant with one of the more unusual varieties of spina bifida aperta lesions such as the asymmetrical lower limb paralysis (Type 6) associated with the hemi-myeloschisis (Figs. 3.1*f* and 6.6), the spastic paraparesis associated with a superficial thoracic or thoraco-lumbar lesion (Type 5), or the spina bifida lesions surmounted by a subcutaneous lipoma or abnormal hair-bearing skin which is closely related to the spina bifida occulta group (see Chapter 7). This is an important group with good neurological function which is likely to deteriorate if the spina bifida lesion is not covered by normal skin.

Group E

The puny infant with any of the above lesions complicated by other congenital abnormalities of the cardiovascular, respiratory, gastro-intestinal or genito-urinary systems. In this class the prognosis depends upon the sum of the various mal-formations; if the spina bifida lesion itself has a good prognosis and the associated malformation is treatable, then the prognosis on the whole is good if both can be treated sequentially and successfully. A severe spina bifida lesion and untreatable severe malformations of another system makes the prognosis very poor.

Group F

A puny infant with a spina bifida lesion accompanied by a profound neurological deficit which has been enhanced by associated birth trauma and hypoxia. The basic neurological reflexes are depressed, hypothermia is common, the spinal lesion is usually a myeloschisis or a frank lumbar myelomeningocele, and the lower limbs manifest clinically a lower motor neurone lesion at the time of examination. In this group, the prognosis for survival of the major surgical treatment required to close the spina bifida lesion is poor, and the ultimate general neurological function is also likely to be poor if the cerebral trauma is severe.

The clinical assessment and likely prognosis may then be discussed with the parents, and it is usual to discuss surgical treatment at this stage also (often in conjunction with the paediatrician, see Chapter 12), since the optimal time for closure of these open spina bifida lesions is within twenty-four hours of birth. Immediate closure is recommended for those patients in groups A, B and D, and patients in category E would only be treated if all of the congenital malformations have a relatively good prognosis and the infant can withstand the surgical procedures. Infants in category F should be observed over twenty-four hours in an incubator; if respiratory pattern, temperature control and general neurological function remain poor then operation should not be undertaken, but if they improve to the level of being more or less normal, then the infant should be treated in the appropriate group A to E.

Group C is the difficult group; the robust infant has a high paraplegia with no hip flexion, and mental retardation is likely if hydrocephalus is already present at birth (Lorber 1971). It seems reasonable not to treat these infants surgically, and certainly not to do so if there is an associated congenital kyphus. When there is a low thoracic paraplegia without a kyphus, and without established hydrocephalus at birth, then surgical treatment might be offered if the parents understand and accept the future of managing a totally paraplegic and incontinent child.

Surgical Management

When surgical closure is undertaken, it is best done under general anaesthesia with endotracheal intubation and in a warm operating theatre. Intravenous anaesthesia (ketamine) does not permit maintenance of adequate respiration when drainage of CSF from the operative site may cause brainstem displacement and apnoea. Local anaesthesia does not relax the adjacent muscles sufficiently for good positioning of the back and successful closure of the lesion, and it also causes a predisposition to oedema around the wound.

Intravenous infusion should be commenced pre-operatively and this can conveniently be done through the umbilical vein in the newborn. It is advisable to have blood cross-matched and ready even for the smallest spina bifida aperta lesion, and to replace all blood loss greater than a measured 30ccs.

The infant is placed in the prone position and raised from the operating table by a square sponge-rubber support, with a hole under the chest and abdomen to permit easy breathing and warming by irradiation and convection of the exposed ventral surface of the infant from a warming blanket which underlies the sponge-rubber support. This position permits easy placement of the head for the convenience of managing the endotracheal tube, and easy observation of the perineum and legs during the operative procedure in order to watch for any movement elicited from exposed neural tissues. The rectal temperature is monitored throughout the procedure.

The closure consists of a careful dissection and isolation of the neural tissue in the centre of the sac until its continuity with the spinal cord and nerve roots has been clearly identified. All of this tissue is preserved, and around it a layer is dissected up from the everted pedicles of the vertebrae and paraspinous muscles to produce a cover for the plaque and nerve roots. This cover is termed a 'dural sac' because it is continuous with the dura around the spinal cord on the rostral side of the lesion. The skin is closed after generous undermining in the correct layer as far as necessary in all directions, and although there may be some degree of tension in the wound, this is taken on the stitches in the subcutaneous fascial layer rather than on the skin edge itself (Zachary 1966). Skin grafts are not usually required. A firm gauze dressing is placed over the wound and then this is sealed off from the anus by waterproof strapping.

Post-Operative Management

Post-operatively the infant is nursed prone and care is taken to keep faeces and urine away from the dressing over the wound. The sutures are removed on the tenth day unless there is leakage beforehand; in the latter case the wound is inspected and if there is a CSF leak emergency treatment of hydrocephalus is undertaken. Wounds with necrosis or with primary or secondary infection are treated by drainage, debridement, and then allowed to heal by secondary intention. Late split thickness grafting is resorted to occasionally in these cases.

Bladder care in the post-operative period involves frequent Credé manoeuvres (after every feed) and intermittent catheterisation if the bladder becomes distended. Prophylactic antibiotics are not given, although the wound is cleaned well at the time of operative closure and dusted with neomycin bacitracin spray. Hydrocephalus may be diagnosed and require surgical treatment at any stage in the first three or four weeks (see Chapter 8) and it is customary during this period to obtain baseline assessment of the urinary tract and primary treatment of any fixed congenital deformities of the lower limbs (see Chapters 9, 10 and 11).

Medical Management of the Spinal Lesion

When, for the reasons outlined already, surgical closure of the spinal lesion is not undertaken, management should be along a line designed to avoid the impression of callousness on the one hand, and unnatural preservation of the abnormal situation on the other. It is customary to leave the spina bifida aperta lesion exposed, to nurse the infant in an ordinary cot rather than an incubator, to feed on demand, and not to give prophylactic antibiotics. Irritability in the child can be controlled by a small amount of regular sedation, and a full, compassionate response made to any interest which the parents may wish to show in the infant at this stage. When nursed in this manner it is unusual for these infants with the severe deformities to survive for more than a few weeks.

CHAPTER 7

Assessment and Management of Infants and Children with Spina Bifida Occulta Lesions

Presentation as Dermal Abnormality over Spina Bifida Occulta with or without Associated Diastematomyelia

These children present because the parents notice either a hairy tuft in the sacral region, or a swelling covered with abnormal and sometimes pigmented skin. Direct enquiry or examination may reveal an accompanying neurological deficit either as a sphincter abnormality, a lower motor neurone deficit affecting one limb, or a spastic paraparesis which may be accompanied by pain in the back on movement, and sometimes a radicular lesion referable to the level of the spina bifida occulta. The dermal abnormality may be a disfiguring long tuft of hair, or a symmetrical or asymmetrical soft swelling which is fixed deeply and may or may not be fixed to the skin. This swelling is transilluminable and sometimes increases with coughing or decreases when the patient lies down, indicating that within the lipomatous mass there is also a meningocele in continuity with the subarachnoid space of the spinal canal (see Fig. 7.1).

Presentation as Dermal Sinus with or without Infection

The dermal sinus runs from the lower sacral region upwards, and is of pathological significance if it is deeper than the common sacral dimple which is found in many normal children (Fig. 7.2). In many cases the sinus reaches the spinal dura mater. The sinus may discharge squamous material and become locally infected, as a variety of pilonidal cyst; but the most serious complication is that of meningitis, because the site of invasion by the organism may so easily be overlooked. Gentle probing shows that the sinus goes deeply, and neither this investigation nor the injection of radio-opaque material into the sinus are of much help.

Presentation as 'Orthopaedic Syndrome' (see Chapter 9)

The child presents with a limp and on examination has one leg which is usually smaller than the other and may have an associated talipes deformity. Examination will nearly always reveal some cutaneous or obvious covered bony abnormality of the lumbo-sacral region and the limb shows evidence of a long-standing lower motor neurone lesion (Fig 7.3) (James and Lassman 1960).

Presentation as Abnormality of Sphincters (see Chapter 11)

One of the important causes of incontinence, increased frequency of micturition, and recurrent urinary tract infections in childhood is an occult abnormality of the spine with some terminal myelodysplasia and impairment of the neurological control of the bladder function. The child may have mild stress incontinence, true incontinence with nocturnal enuresis, or may return to incontinence after having been toilet trained. Increased frequency may be associated with dysuria and on examining the urinary tract the commonest finding is a dilated flaccid bladder with or without hydronephrosis; in a few cases with diastematomyelia the bladder is spastic, contracted and may have diverticula. Again, the spinal abnormality may be suspected on clinical examination of the overlying skin.

Radiological Diagnosis of Abnormalities Associated with Spina Bifida Occulta

Straight X-rays of the spine will reveal the increased interpedicular distance associated with a spina bifida, and the actual site is usually in the sacral or lower lumbar region. In addition, the outline of midline bony spurs which accompany diastematomyelia at the level of the spina bifida occulta or higher will also be shown in the plain radiographs of the spine (Fig. 7.4). The lateral views will sometimes show an increased anteroposterior diameter of the spinal canal, with scalloping of the vertebral bodies which may accompany an intraspinal lipoma or dermoid, or merely accompany the abnormally large subarachnoid space which is sometimes a feature of these developmental abnormalities. These specific radiological features distinguish the condition from the sacral spina bifida occulta which is unaccompanied by neurological abnormalities and is a common finding in the normal population.

A myelogram with radio-opaque dye ('Myodil' or 'Pantopaque') will often confirm the enlarged spinal canal and outline any midline spur which accompanies diastematomyelia (see Fig. 7.5). Sometimes the upper end of an intraspinal lipoma will also be outlined, but the technique of myelography in the presence of spina bifida

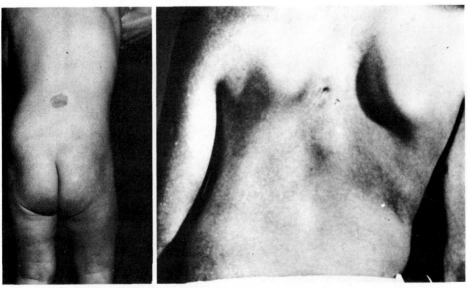

Fig. 7.1 (*left*). Spina bifida occulta with pigmented abnormal skin overlying diastematomyelia. (Photograph by courtesy of Dr. Lloyd Megison, Jr.)
Fig. 7.2 (*right*). Spina bifida occulta with dermal sinus and underlying diastematomyelia. (Photograph by courtesy of Dr. Lloyd Megison, Jr.)

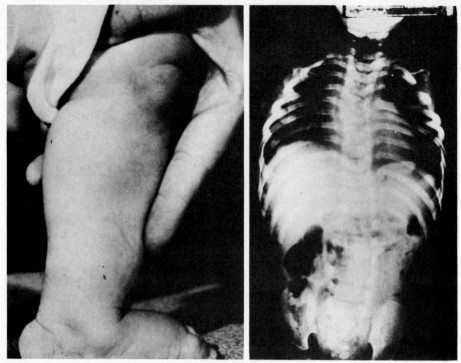

Fig. 7.3 (*left*). The orthopaedic syndrome with spina bifida occulta and diastematomyelia with spur (see Fig. 9.7 and Ch. 9).
Fig. 7.4 (*right*). Spina bifida occulta with diastematomyelia. Straight radiograph of spine. (Photographs by courtesy of Dr. Lloyd Megison, Jr.)

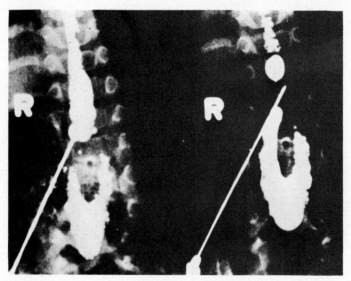

Fig. 7.5. Spina bifida occulta and diastematomyelia with bony spur; myelogram. (Photograph by courtesy of Dr. Lloyd Megison, Jr.)

66

and a lipoma is often difficult. In such cases, a high lateral cervical puncture may have to be performed and the dye run downwards from the cervical region. In many centres, air myelography has been satisfactorily performed in infants with these lesions; the air is injected usually through the lumbar route, but sometimes through the lateral cervical route, and the pictures are obtained by lateral tomography. This technique blurs the bones and outlines the spinal cord, and will often demonstrate the level of the conus medullaris and the myelodysplasia or other lesions in the region of the spina bifida occulta.

Management of Spinal Lesions in Association with Spina Bifida Occulta, and When to Operate

Clearly, a sinus that may lead to intraspinal and intracranial infection should be excised as soon as it comes to clinical attention, even if this is in the neonatal period. After the appropriate clinical and radiological investigations have been carried out, the surgeon should trace the sinus down to the dura through the spina bifida occulta and then open the dura and explore the spinal canal for any other abnormality. A water-tight dural repair should then be performed.

The disfiguring hairy tuft overlying a spina bifida occulta lesion can be treated, on purely plastic or cosmetic grounds, by a plastic surgical procedure. However, as radical excision of the skin may inadvertently open up the spinal canal, more simple epilation methods are preferable.

In other respects, treatment of spina bifida occulta with accompanying lipomatous abnormalities should be approached in the same way as that of diastematomyelia: if there is undoubted evidence of an increasing neurological deficit, particularly if it is a spastic paraparesis, or increasing sphincter problems, then the lesion should be explored, the lipomatous masses excised, large midline spurs carefully removed, and every care taken to avoid dissection into the conus medullaris itself. Prophylactic excision of these lesions has been advised on the basis that neurological deterioration is related to trauma and vascular impairment around these lesions, and sometimes to the actual compressive effect of a lipomatous mass or dermoid. However, there is little definite proof that such undertakings lead to neurological improvement; the neurological position can often remain unchanged after surgical treatment, as is also the case when no intervention is undertaken.

In general, since the risk of increasing the neurological lesion is small if surgical treatment is undertaken with a neurosurgical technique and using the dissecting microscope, it is probably justified in the majority of cases (James and Lassman 1964, 1967, 1972; Guthkelch 1974).

CHAPTER 8

Assessment and Management of Hydrocephalus

Diagnosis of Hydrocephalus in the Neonatal Period

The diagnosis of hydrocephalus in infants with spina bifida lesions is most simply made on clinical grounds; observations of the general behaviour of the child, fontanelle tension and skull circumference should lead to an early diagnosis in the neonatal period (see Fig. 8.1). Using a soft tape, the skull circumference is measured in a plane just above the orbits and incorporating the most protruberant part of the occiput. A chart (see Fig. 8.2) is used to provide the normal range of skull circumference related to the age of the infant, and should include that of premature births. It is also useful to compare the skull circumference with the chest circumference, since these two measurements normally agree within one centimetre for the first few months of life. In this way an impression may be confirmed that an apparently normal skull circumference for a particular age of a child is actually too large for that child's size, or, on the other hand, an apparently large circumference is quite normal because the size of the child is also large for its particular age.

Serial measurements are also useful, for when a skull circumference moves from being well below the 50th percentile to above it over a short period of time, it is unnecessary to wait for it to exceed the 90th percentile before diagnosing hydrocephalus.

It should be noted that in some cases hydrocephalus develops acutely in a relatively normal shaped head and before the circumference significantly increases. This type of hydrocephalus may occur in infants with low sacral myelomeningoceles and no evidence of craniodysplasia (see Chapter 4); the slight ventricular enlargement in the presence of a well-preserved cerebral cortex causes acutely raised pressure and apnoea may rapidly supervene. In some cases there may be a persistant CSF fistula through the wound over the spina bifida, and in others hydrocephalus may develop very slowly and may not be apparent until the patient is reviewed in an out-patient clinic two to three months after the spinal operation.

Additional procedures

Confirmation of hydrocephalus may be made either by demonstrating ventricular enlargement at the time of operation, or, if there is a reasonable doubt, an air ventriculogram may be undertaken. This radiographic investigation, performed by puncture of the ventricles through the lateral angle of the anterior fontanelle, is preceded by the slow decompression of the ventricular system and the injection of 10ccs of air for the initial 'scout' films; these give some idea of ventricular size, cortical thickness, and the amount of air which will be required to give good filling of the ventricular system. Thereafter, fractional replacement of CSF with air is undertaken until the injected air escapes from the contra-lateral intraventricular needle; brow-up pictures taken at this stage will demonstrate the patency of the interventricular foramina and the position of the anterior third ventricle. A backward somersault to the brow-down position will probably catch enough air in the posterior third ventricle to outline this structure as well as the occipital horns of the lateral ventricles. Demonstration of the fourth ventricle and cisterna magna will be obtained by taking pictures with the child inverted, provided that the aqueduct is patent. Outlining basal cisterns and the temporal horns may be achieved by returning the infant to the brow-up position. The whole procedure may be performed with carbon dioxide gas instead of air, and since the former is absorbed more rapidly, a ventriculo-atrial shunt procedure can be undertaken directly following the investigation, without the risk of air embolus via the shunt tubing.

Contrast ventriculography, using 60 per cent 'Conray' diluted with CSF or saline is an entirely satisfactory procedure provided that the amount of 'Conray' injected is directly related to the estimate of ventricular size obtained through the 'scout' films; a grossly enlarged ventricular system requires 8 to 10ccs of dye to avoid excessive dilution of the contrast and failure to outline the third ventricle, and small ventricles require only 5ccs to avoid the escape of contrast over the cerebellum and up to the cerebral convexities which gives rise to serious decerebrate spasms.

Lumbar air studies (pneumoencephalography) are of rather limited value as it is sometimes technically difficult to introduce air satisfactorily above the spina bifida lesions due to the abnormally low spinal cord; furthermore, the air may merely outline the brainstem malformation and never enter the ventricular system at all if the obstruction is at the level of the foramen magnum or fourth ventricle itself. On the other hand, air studies have been used to outline the central canal which can usually be catheterised directly through the plaque of a frank myeloschisis; the position of the fourth ventricle and an outline of the lateral ventricles may be obtained in this manner, provided that the central canal does actually communicate with the fourth ventricle.

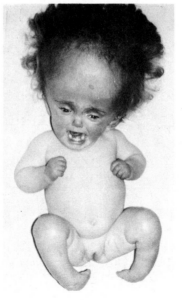

Fig. 8.1. Advanced hydrocephalus in infant with untreated spina bifida aperta lesion.

'Myodil' ventriculography is the least satisfactory of investigations because the heavy contrast medium easily gets lost in the large ventricles unless it is injected in such a manner that it drops straightaway into the dilated third ventricle, when it can be satisfactorily manipulated backwards and used to give a very accurate outline of the brainstem malformation.

Computerised axial tomography (E.M.I. scanner) is a most reliable way of demonstrating ventricular enlargement, and is minimally disturbing to the patient; with increasing availability of this facility, most other methods of investigation are likely to be superceded.

Manometric readings at the time of the ventricular puncture may show that the pressure is raised, but owing to the many variable factors in the generation of intracranial pressure in the neonatal period, a single manometer reading is unsatisfactory. More accurate pressure recordings are obtained by using a pressure transducer which is attached to an intraventricular needle or a subcutaneous reservoir continuous with an intraventricular catheter (the reservoir can be tapped by inserting a sharp needle through the scalp). In the newborn infant with its soft head, the intracranial pressure (using the position of the interventricular foramen as a baseline) should be under 10mm of mercury in the brow-up position. Pressure readings should

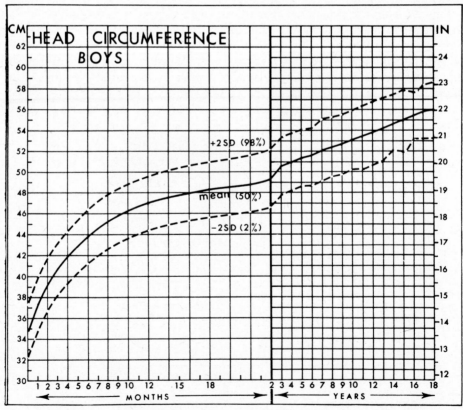

Fig. 8.2 (and see facing page). Head circumference charts (from Dr. G. Nellhaus, 1968).

be continued for an hour or more until the infant is relatively quiet, when the record should show the small variations in intracranial pressure with each cardiac impulse and respiratory cycle. These variations are enhanced when the baseline pressure is raised.

Isotope ventriculography, using 50 microcuries of radio-iodinated human serum albumin, is of some value in the diagnosis of hydrocephalus; it gives an indication of the bulk-flow of CSF over the course of 24 to 48 hours, and when the tracer does not leave the ventricular system during that time there is little doubt about the diagnosis. However, when the somewhat varied patterns are analysed, interpretation is often difficult and the investigation may ultimately prove to be more useful in confirming arrested hydrocephalus than progressive hydrocephalus (Brocklehurst 1968*b*, Front *et al.* 1972).

On the whole, the demonstration of ventricular dilatation in an infant can be considered indicative of hydrocephalus when it is accompanied by the clinical features of that condition, or by abnormally high pressure readings, or is shown by repeated contrast studies to be progressive. On the other hand, enlargement of the ventricular system alone may not be of much diagnostic value, since it is the usual consequence of any destructive brain process (such as that following trauma, cerebrovascular lesions, or intracranial infection).

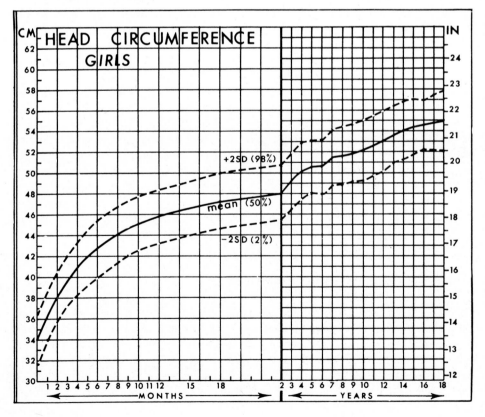

Medical Treatment of Hydrocephalus

Ninety per cent of infants with spina bifida aperta lesions have some degree of brainstem malformation. When routine ventriculography is performed in the neonatal period, the majority of these infants will show ventricular enlargement, although relatively few have an abnormal skull circumference at this stage (Lorber 1961). Some 10 to 15 per cent of these infants will not require surgical treatment as the condition does not progress to a level of clinical significance and there is no mental impairment in later life.

In an effort to decrease the proportion of infants with progressive hydrocephalus who require an operation, various attempts have been made in recent years to treat these infants by medical means. The effect of acetazolamide upon the production of cerebrospinal fluid in man (acting as a carbonic anhydrase inhibitor on the choroid plexus) proved too brief to avert hydrocephalus in infants with spina bifida aperta lesions (Huttenlocher 1965, Ruben *et al.* 1966, Mealey and Barker 1968). Isosorbide (1, 4: 3, 6 Dianhydro-D-Glucitol) is an osmotic agent which has been presented for clinical use as a 45 per cent solution under the name of 'Hydranol'; its effect in reducing intracranial pressure associated with hydrocephalus was described by Hayden and Shurtleff in 1967. They found, by measuring intraventricular pressure, that an effective dose was somewhere between 2.5 to 3g/kg given at intervals of 6 to 12 hours, and in 1972 they reported its use in a series of trials on patients with hydrocephalus. The short-term results showed control of ventricular pressure and also of the increasing skull circumference, but this was less satisfactory over periods extending into weeks; not only were there episodes of hypernatraemia and increase of blood urea nitrogen but it was clear both from the clinical and animal experiments that body dehydration had to be maintained to avoid a renewed rise in intracranial pressure. Lorber, using the same drug at a dosage of 2g/kg bodyweight every six hours over three weeks, showed a prolonged effect in controlling hydrocephalus (as judged by skull circumference measurements and repeated ventriculography), provided that the cortical thickness was 20mm or greater, *i.e.* patients with extreme hydrocephalus and a cortical thickness of 14mm or thereabouts did not show a maintained response and were subjected to surgical treatment. The side-effects of this osmotic, diuretic type of therapy are also clear from these trials, and the combination of hypernatraemia and renal uremia with impaired renal function may occur (Lorber 1972, 1973*b*). The place of such medical therapy of hydrocephalus is therefore limited and requires careful monitoring, particularly if sudden rises of intracranial pressure accompanied by irreversible neurological sequelae are to be avoided.

Surgical Treatment of Neonatal Hydrocephalus

Whenever hydrocephalus is clinically progressive (as judged by abnormally increased skull circumference, persistently increased anterior fontanelle tension, episodes of respiratory slowing, apnoea, or decerebration, or a persistent CSF fistula from a lumbar wound) then surgical treatment should be undertaken without delay. In difficult cases, the additional diagnostic procedures described above should be undertaken.

When hydrocephalus is already manifest at the time of birth (by abnormally increased skull circumference), the infant should not be treated surgically unless a decision has already been made to prolong the life of a child with severe mental retardation; particularly when the hydrocephalus is accompanied by brilliant transillumination of the cranial vault and radiological demonstration of a cortical thickness of 5mm or less.

In a straightforward situation, *i.e.* with increased skull circumference and clear CSF obtained at the time of ventricular puncture, the operation of choice is a shunting procedure from the ventricular system to the atrium or peritoneal cavity. The ventriculo-atrial shunt using the Pudenz-Heyer or Holter type of valve is quite satisfactory in the neonatal period, although blockage of the lower end of such a shunt by the time the infant is nine months of age is almost inevitable; normal growth causes retraction of the tip of the catheter from the atrium (where the turbulent blood flow keeps it unblocked) to the superior vena cava or innominate vein, where laminar flow permits the walling-off of the tip of the tube. For this reason, many surgeons will perform a ventriculo-peritoneal shunt as the first procedure, and, when this blocks, will do the ventriculo-atrial shunt at a time when the child is a little older. The further details of shunt management are discussed below.

Hydrocephalus in Children after Infancy

The clinical manifestations of progressive hydrocephalus in an older infant or child are various and sometimes difficult to define. By the age of 18 months the membranous bones of the skull usually interdigitate sufficiently along the sutures to prevent any rapid increase of skull circumference as a response to raised intracranial pressure and ventricular dilatation; the small amount of suture spreading which does occur may only be detected by a lateral skull X-ray in which the coronal suture can be seen, and this should not exceed 2mm in width at the age of three years. The percussion note is also sometimes abnormal and likened to a cracked pot when hydrocephalus occurs within the firmer cranial vault of the older child. In some cases there may be a classical history of raised intracranial pressure, *viz.* complaints of headache and vomiting, particularly in the early morning. These bouts of intracranial hypertension may be intermittent and can easily be precipitated by an intercurrent infection or by minimal skull trauma. Papilloedema may or may not accompany this more classical syndrome, depending a little upon whether there has been previous papilloedema and secondary optic atrophy. In some cases the clinical symptoms may be lacking but the papilloedema striking, and in other cases the effect of the chronically raised intracranial pressure upon the optic discs is to produce progressive secondary atrophy and increasing blindness.

The appearance or reappearance of a squint due either to a VIth-nerve palsy or to an enhancement of a congenital esophoria may be an indication of hydrocephalus in an older child. Quite often the clinical symptoms are completely lacking, but the parents report that the child has slipped back in motor or mental progress and has become more irritable in behaviour.

There is a small but important group of children with previously treated hydrocephalus which has been followed by some abnormal degree of premature fusion of the sutures and a resultant craniostenosis (usually scaphocephalic or plagiocephalic in shape). The recurrence of hydrocephalus in these children can be dramatic and accompanied by grossly raised intracranial pressure with secondary brainstem disturbance such as decerebrate attacks (so-called 'cerebellar fit') or sudden apnoea. Another small group includes children with more subtle brainstem reflex disturbances such as episodes of pallor, sweating, or flushing of the head, neck and upper trunk, and these phenomena occur more commonly in those patients with high, severe spina bifida lesions, pre-existing ventricular dilatation, and gross congenital brainstem malformation.

These older children with episodes of recurrent hydrocephalus require considerable clinical experience and caution in their management if the catastrophe of sudden unconsciousness, apnoea, and death is to be avoided. A general rule is to pay great attention to any complaints or symptoms related by the parents, and to admit the children for hospital observation on the least suspicion. Access to the ventricular system via the reservoir of a shunt apparatus (see below) is of great help both for diagnostic procedures and emergency treatment, and familiarity with these devices is important (see Fig. 8.3). A single pressure reading (if greatly raised) will be sufficient to confirm the situation, but in some cases repeated contrast ventriculography, continuous intracranial pressure recordings, and isotope ventriculography may be required.

Technique of primary shunting procedures

The surgical technique of the insertion of these shunts should include meticulous attention to skin cleansing and the avoidance of contact of the various tubes with the skin during the operation. It is preferable to establish the position of the ventricular catheter first (*i.e.* before doing the cardiac end of the shunt); the ventricle is then customarily approached through a small posterior temporal burr-hole beneath a small scalp flap on the right side of the head. The catheter should be run obliquely into the ventricle so that it lies along the body of the ventricle towards the frontal horn or interventricular foramen; there should be about 4cm of the catheter within the ventricle. Before attaching the ventricular catheter to a reservoir, CSF should be running freely through it. The catheter is attached to the underside of the reservoir and the junction ligated. The reservoir (which may be entirely of 'Silastic' and contain various diaphragms and inner chambers to facilitate its use for diagnosis and therapy, or just a simple chamber with a metal underside as in the Rickham type—see Fig. 8.3) is sutured into position within the burr-hole in the skull, and the side-arm is temporarily closed off so that excessive drainage of CSF does not occur.

It is customarily assumed that the right side of the head and neck is the best for the initial shunting procedure because, compared with the left side, the course of the internal jugular vein down to the innominate vein and superior vena cava is in a fairly straight line. Entry to the internal jugular vein is usually obtained by identifying the facial vein just beneath the angle of the mandible, and if this tributary is large enough, the catheter can be inserted into it using a controlling ligature. The catheter is then filled with saline and used as an ECG electrode; it is passed down until the recorded P-wave is biphasic, which leaves the tip in the mid-atrium (Brocklehurst *et al.* 1967c). The cardiac catheter is then ligated into the facial or internal jugular vein, and the upper end tunnelled under the skin and joined and ligated to the side-arm of the reservoir.

In the Pudenz-Heyer type of shunt, the non-return valve (which permits CSF drainage and prevents blood regurgitating into the ventricular system) is a little slit valve situated at the tip of the cardiac catheter (see Fig. 8.3); in the Spitz-Holter shunt, the valve is a little cartridge situated subcutaneously just below the site of the insertion of the ventricular catheter at the side of the head. In both cases the catheter is tested for the hydrostatic column which it will support before it opens; this should be around 50 to 70mm of saline for the usual shunting procedure. Valves with a lower closing pressure may be used if it is anticipated that the intraventricular pressure may not be greatly raised, such as in hydrocephalus of a more indolent type or in those patients with gross ventricular dilatation.

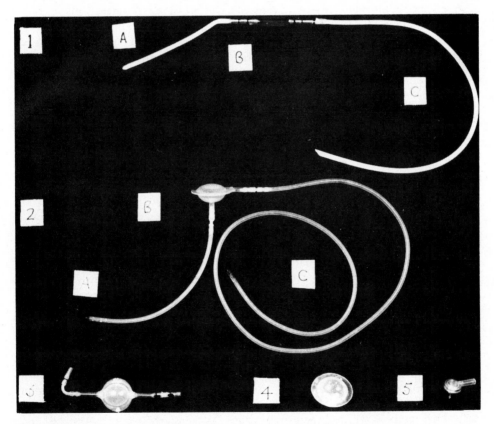

Fig. 8.3. Various shunt devices.
1. Spitz Holter shunt. A—ventricular catheter. B—valve. C—cardiac catheter.
2. Pudenz-Heyer shunt. A—ventricular catheter. B—reservoir. C—cardiac catheter (with valve at tip).
3. Foltz reservoir.
4. Mishler double-lumen reservoir.
5. Rickham reservoir (with side-arm).

In the ventriculo-peritoneal shunt the catheter which is inserted into the peritoneal cavity through a right upper quadrant incision is reinforced with coiled wire to prevent its occlusion by pressure of the abdominal contents or muscles (the Raimondi catheter). It is burrowed under the skin and joined to the side-arm of the reservoir of the ventricular catheter in the same manner as in the ventriculo-atrial shunts. The Raimondi catheter has a slit valve at its tip, with an opening pressure similar to that of the atrial catheters. CSF drainage occurs through these valves only when the intraventricular pressure is somewhere in excess of 50mm of saline, which is considerably less than half of the accepted upper level of normal (*i.e.* 10mm of mercury).

Post-operatively the infants are nursed supine or sitting up if a little older, and the effectiveness of the shunt can be easily ascertained by inspection of the fontanelles and sutures which will rapidly become slack and infallen. On the fifth day the wounds are inspected, the sutures removed and the reservoir can be tested by simple compression, but it should not require routine compression post-operatively since the well-functioning valvular system opens by the excess of hydrostatic pressure and not by using the reservoir as a pump. Indeed, there is some danger that excessive pumping of a reservoir may so collapse the ventricular system that the ventricular catheter impinges upon the choroid plexus or ventricular wall, and these structures are sucked up into its lumen which then becomes occluded.

Post-operative X-rays of the skull and chest confirm the position of the tips of the catheters and form a baseline for future observations should there be any question of catheter blockage or detachment of the various pieces of the shunt.

Shunt devices

The shunt devices most commonly used in surgical practice are illustrated in Fig. 8.3. The basic difference in siting of the valve in the Pudenz-Heyer type and the Spitz-Holter type has already been described. The simplest reservoirs consist of a chamber with two ducts and no diaphragm within the chamber. The Rickham type has one duct composed of metal as part of the underside of the shunt, and another duct leading from the side of the 'Silastic' cap. Palpation or compression of such a reservoir gives little information because it is so small, but it can easily be tapped through the skin, and, provided that the ventricular catheter is not occluded, CSF from the ventricular system can be obtained for both chemical and bacterial analysis, and at the same time a single pressure reading can be taken. If the two ends of the shunt are patent, direct injection into such a reservoir will enter both the ventricular system and the heart or peritoneal cavity, and in this way an infected shunt can be treated with local antibiotics. The Foltz reservoir is of similarly simple design except that the whole of it is made of 'Silastic' and the arms come from the side. By pressing one arm the ventricular catheter can be occluded from the system and a compression test of the reservoir will test the atrial end; or, alternatively, by occluding the other arm directly a compression test of the ventricular catheter can be made. Similarly, the tapping of the reservoir combined with compression of one or other side-arms determines the sampling and injection of any fluid.

The commonly used Schulte reservoir has a slack diaphragm across it and in an ordinarily functioning shunt CSF comes into the bottom of the chamber, passes through the holes in the side of the diaphragm and then out of the side-arm to drain into the heart, depending upon hydrostatic pressure and the closing pressure of the slit valve. On compression of such a reservoir the diaphragm is forced downwards to exclude the ventricular component of the shunt and the fluid in the chamber is pushed out of the side-arm and through the cardiac catheter. If the ventricular catheter is patent, the chamber will quickly re-fill when the finger is released; by repeating this manoeuvre once or twice the patency of the ventricular end, and the ease with which fluid can be forced through the atrial end can be judged. When the atrial end is completely blocked then the chamber of this particular reservoir does not compress. Tapping of such a reservoir will only obtain a significant quantity of CSF if the ventricular catheter is patent, and similarly a pressure reading will be obtained in the same circumstances. Injection into the Schulte chamber will not go into the ventricular system but will go straight down the side-arm and into the atrium. Various double-lumen reservoirs are in use and are designed to obtain diagnostic information about both ends of the catheter and to permit sampling and injection in both directions.

The Denver shunt and the Hakim shunt have a cartridge form similar to the Spitz-Holter device but have different mechanical and hydraulic features.

It must be acknowledged that none of these shunts has hydraulic properties sufficiently adaptable to reproduce the normal physiological CSF system (although see discussion by Hakim 1973).

Alternative operative procedures—internal shunts

The possibility of treating hydrocephalus by operative procedures that restore the normal physiology of the cerebrospinal fluid is attractive, and also has the advantage of avoiding the many complications of the external shunting procedures. The increased evidence of the co-existence of an actual or potential subarachnoid space in many infants and children with hydrocephalus has encouraged this approach (see Chapter 3).

The Torkildsen procedure consists of a shunt from the occipital horn of the lateral ventricle to the cisterna magna by a tube which runs underneath or within a groove of the occipital bone. It is well established as a treatment for straightforward aqueduct stenosis, but is obviously unsuitable for a condition in which the cisterna magna is occupied by the malformed brainstem.

Third ventriculostomy enables CSF to drain directly from the third ventricle to the basal cisterns, and has been recently modified by Brocklehurst (1974a), using the trans-callosal approach to the third ventricle. This procedure, termed 'trans-callosal third ventriculo-chiasmatic cisternostomy,' has met with some limited success and more attention to these internal shunting procedures may be ultimately rewarding.

Various modifications of the external shunting procedures have been made, and the CSF has been diverted to nearly every possible site in the body, from the mastoid air cells to the ureters; but none of these procedures has stood the test of time compared with the ventriculo-atrial and ventriculo-peritoneal shunts.

A useful addition to the shunting procedures is that of the 'false fontanelle'

(Forrest and Tsingoglou 1968). The value of the open fontanelle as a means of assessing intracranial pressure in infancy is well known to all clinicians, but after the age of 18 months this is not available. In these older hydrocephalic children a false fontanelle is made at the parietal eminence, where, through a large burr-hole, dural substitute is sutured in place and remains patent for a year or more.

Shunt complications

These are various and frequent. The summarised experience shows a 46 per cent complication rate, a six per cent mortality and a 66 per cent arrest of hydrocephalus (Scarff 1963). Hemmer (1967) reported a 62 per cent revision rate in a series of 181 infants where both Holter and Pudenz types of valve were used; he noted that 44 per cent of revisions were for problems with the ventricular catheter and 55 per cent with the cardiac catheter. The infection rate was ten per cent and complications due to thrombosis around the cardiac catheter nine per cent. He noted that 65 per cent of the revisions took place within six months of insertion of the shunt, and only nine of them at the end of the second year. Forrest *et al.* (1966) reported an infection rate of 15.8 per cent and, from their studies, concluded that most of the shunts had been revised by the fourth aniversary of the insertion and that 26 per cent had been revised by the end of the first year. Most of these complications are related to the use of a relatively rigid tubular system with a set opening-pressure of the valve in a situation beset with physiological variables, including that of growth. In addition, there is the association of an intravascular foreign body with persistent infection by organisms derived from the skin at the time of the initial operation, or derived from infected sites elsewhere in the body. A very meticulous surgical technique can considerably reduce the incidence of complications but cannot eliminate them entirely.

The ventriculo-peritoneal shunt, when first performed, had a higher incidence of complications due to blockage than did the ventriculo-atrial shunts; but more recently, by using the specially designed catheters and placing a good length within the peritoneal cavity, lower-end blockage has been reduced. The absence of septicaemia with this type of shunt is offset by the occurrence of intra-abdominal complications such as low grade peritonitis and bowel obstruction.

Detached shunts

The junctions of the various parts of the shunt are customarily secured with a silk ligature at the time of the operation, but they nevertheless frequently become detached; the cardiac end then migrates down the inferior vena cava or through the ventricles of the heart and into the lungs, and the upper end of the shunt falls into the lateral ventricle or third ventricle. When a shunt becomes detached there is a transitory accumulation of CSF beneath the skin around the reservoir, and, when this has been later walled-off, the palpatory findings are similar to those of a blocked shunt. It is of considerable value in these circumstances to compare skull X-rays and chest or abdominal X-rays with the immediate post-operative pictures.

Blockage of the ventricular catheter

This occurs almost as frequently as blockage of the distal end of the shunt, but it is usually more acute and occurs somewhat sooner after the insertion. It is due to the tip of the ventricular catheter sucking in choroid plexus, ependymal lining of the ventricles and brain, or blood clot. It is more likely if the ventricular catheter is rather long and the tip is well towards the frontal horn or temporal horns, and it is particularly likely to occur when the shunt has been performed for high pressure hydrocephalus at a stage before massive ventricular enlargement. When the operation is undertaken at this early stage, the relief of the hydrocephalus permits the brain to re-expand; the ventricles become relatively normal in size so that the tube is impinged upon quite rapidly by ependyma or choroid plexus. A sequence of recurrent obstruction occurs with acute clinical deterioration each time, emergency revision, and then the repeat of the whole process. When the ventricular catheter is blocked, compression of the reservoir which contains a diaphragm (see above and Fig. 8.3) will empty the reservoir and then it will not fill.

Blockage of the cardiac catheter

When the distal tip of a ventriculo-atrial shunt is situated in the atrium it is surrounded by blood with turbulent flow and does not become easily occluded; but when the tip is situated in a great vein such as the superior vena cava or innominate vein, then laminar flow occurs, and in these circumstances the emerging CSF produces a slow reaction and the tip of the shunt becomes walled off with fibrin until it is lying in a cul-de-sac. This is the more common mechanism with the Pudenz-Heyer type of shunt, and actual thrombosis of the superior vena cava around the tip of the shunt appears to be more common in the Spitz-Holter where the tip is an open tube. The time after insertion at which blockage of the cardiac catheter occurs depends upon a mixture of the following factors:

(*1*) *The siting of the tip of the catheter at the time of the initial operation.* This may be done by ECG control; the tip is customarily left at the point where the cardiac catheter reads a biphasic P wave, which is mid-atrium (Brocklehurst *et al.* 1967c), or by X-ray control, making the assumption that the atrium is around the level of the eighth thoracic vertebra. When the shunt tip is higher in the atrium it will clearly be a shorter time before growth causes it to reach the superior vena cava, and if shunts are intentionally inserted so low in the atrium that they are in the inferior vena cava there appears to be a higher likelihood of the tip becoming infected.

(*2*) *The age of the infant at the time of insertion.* Growth is much more rapid in the earlier months of infancy, and a shunt in the mid-atrial position at the age of six weeks will reach the superior vena cava by the age of eight months.

(*3*) *The length of time since the shunt was inserted.* While there is growth occurring in the child the position of the lower end of the shunt will continue to move relatively upwards, although this occurs much more slowly as the child gets older.

(*4*) *The actual site where walling-off occurs.* In some cases the cardiac catheter will become obstructed as soon as it is situated in the superior vena cava, and some will remain patent even though the tip is in the internal jugular vein. The reasons for this particular variability are not known. Tsingoglou and Forrest (1968) endeavoured to assess this factor of differential growth by examining the radiographs of patients in whom the shunts had been inserted within the first six weeks of life and were initially in the low atrium. By eight months they had reached the superior vena cava atrial junction, by 12 months were in the low superior vena cava, by 14 months in the mid superior vena cava, and by 20 months in the upper superior vena cava. However, these figures were obtained as averages of a very wide range of numbers, and the final observation that the tip may reach the jugular vein anywhere from 16 months to four years epitomizes the immense variability. In general, it may be said that any catheter lying above the level of the sixth thoracic vertebra may become walled-off, but this is by no means certainly so.

Pulmonary emboli and hypertension

This complication has been described with the Spitz-Holter shunt in a significant number of patients (Erdohazi *et al.* 1966). It consists of the repeated detachment of emboli from the tip of the shunt; these become lodged in the pulmonary circulation and eventually produce pulmonary hypertension and right-heart failure. The pathology of this has been well defined in post-mortem examinations, and the process can be demonstrated in life by performing serial Technetium-99 lung scans.

Shunt infections

These are of relatively common occurrence (around 10 per cent) and may take either an acute or subacute form. The acute form presents in the early post-operative period and is marked by pyrexia, irritability, signs of meningitis, erythema of the wound and septicaemia. The infecting organism is usually a staphylococcus but may be a gram negative organism and the diagnosis is usually confirmed by obtaining CSF from the reservoir of the shunt. In the subacute form, the child may present at any time from a few weeks to months after the shunt has been inserted and is typically irritable, failing to thrive, anaemic and has a low-grade, intermittent pyrexia. Enlargement of the liver and spleen are usually found on examination and there may be haematuria from accompanying nephritis. Confirmation of the diagnosis is obtained by isolating the organism from the reservoir of the shunt and from the blood stream; it is usually a coagulase negative staphylococcus (staphylococcus albus or epidermidis).

General management of shunt complications

The basic principle in the management of shunt complications is to recognise the various clinical entities and to undertake the necessary diagnostic procedures to confirm the clinical diagnosis before the condition has become too advanced.

In some centres the problem of obstruction of the cardiac end of the shunt has been dealt with by undertaking prophylactic revision when the tip of the shunt is at the superior vena cava/atrial junction (sixth thoracic vertebra) on plain radiographs. An analysis of these prophylactic revisions showed the incidence of further complications and the general morbidity and mortality of the operative procedure to be significantly lower than when revision was undertaken as an emergency (Tsingoglou and Forrest 1968). However, in view of the immense variability in the time of occurrence of this complication (*see above*) it seems likely that the decision to perform prophylactic revision on such an arbitrary basis will result in a large number of unnecessary operations. It must also be remembered that obstruction to the cardiac end constitutes only just over 50 per cent of the shunt blockages. Quite often the blockage of a shunt will pass unnoticed because the hydrocephalus has undergone spontaneous arrest and the child is now independent of the shunt (*see below*). In other cases, the recurrence of hydrocephalus may produce anything from the mildest clinical disturbance to the most acute clinical syndrome of rapidly deepening unconsciousness and apnoea. The clinical diagnosis and further investigation of the older child with hydrocephalus has already been discussed.

Treatment of detached shunts

Recurrence of hydrocephalus following detachment of part of a shunt requires a revision of the ventriculo-atrial procedure; in addition to this, if the cardiac catheter has migrated through the heart into the lung or down into the inferior vena cava it should be removed by a direct surgical approach. A ventricular catheter lying loose in the ventricular system should be left where it is.

Treatment of blockage of ventricular catheter

This is diagnosed by palpating and then puncturing the reservoir (using full aseptic technique) to demonstrate that no fluid can be obtained from the ventricles. The situation is confirmed at the operation when the reservoir is exposed. The side-arm is detached and this demonstrates that no CSF flows through the reservoir; the cardiac catheter is clipped off and the reservoir removed, bringing the ventricular catheter with it. This is done gently, for fear of avulsing the choroid plexus and producing an intraventricular haematoma. The blocked ventricular catheter is replaced by a new one with a length calculated to put the tip in the body of the right lateral ventricle. For the syndrome of recurrent upper-end obstruction, a flanged ventricular catheter or ventricular catheter with a small balloon at the tip may be used to keep the ependyma and choroid plexus away from the catheter tip as the ventricle becomes smaller.

Treatment of the blocked cardiac end of the shunt

This operation should be prepared for by obtaining the assistance of an anaesthetist who is expert in managing these situations, and by having an intravenous infusion running at the time of the procedure. Blood should have previously been cross-matched in anticipation of exploration of the neck with the risk of severe venous haemorrhage. The blocked cardiac catheter is confirmed by detaching it from the side-arm of the reservoir and then putting on a manometer filled with saline and seeing that the meniscus level in the manometer does not fall. Syringing through the cardiac catheter may produce a temporary return of drainage, but this usually does not persist satisfactorily. The neck is then opened and the internal jugular vein identified. Occasionally there may still be blood in the internal jugular vein running alongside the fibrous sheath which contains the cardiac catheter, and this is particularly so if the facial vein was used for the initial entry. However, in many cases there is no internal jugular vein and the next direct entry to the heart is the right innominate vein. This is identified by extending the incision down the anterior border of the sternomastoid, detaching the latter muscle from the upper end of the clavicle and tracing the fibrous internal jugular vein down until it is joined by the subclavian to form the innominate. A controlling ligature is placed around the upper end of the innominate vein, and a sufficiently small incision made so as to enable the tip of the shunt to be passed in without losing too much venous blood. Using the ECG monitoring, the hunt is passed easily on to the atrium where it can be localised satisfactorily. The ligature is then tied down on the entry into the innominate vein without occluding the subclavian vein. This procedure is a major undertaking in an infant or small child, and there is the additional risk of opening the pleural cavity over the apex of the lung. By undertaking such a procedure, the transferral of the shunt to the left side of the neck is postponed, and if it is performed on both sides of the neck this permits at least three revisions for a blocked cardiac end. It is very unusual for a child to outgrow a shunt and still require it beyond this stage, because not only does relative growth become less but after the age of five years spontaneous arrest of the hydrocephalus commonly occurs and the child becomes shunt independent. However, if there is no vein left in the neck there should be no hesitation in placing the cardiac catheter through a direct thoracotomy and atriotomy, as described by Blazé *et al.* (1971).

Treatment of shunt thrombosis and pulmonary embolisation

If this complication is suspected it is wise to obtain a venogram (if necessary via the shunt tubing) in order to demonstrate the state of the superior vena cava. If there is superior vena cava occlusion then the shunt should be revised and a direct atriotomy performed. Replacement of a Spitz-Holter by a Pudenz-Heyer shunt may stop the embolisation, particularly if the catheter tip is replaced into the mid-atrium.

Treatment of shunt infections

Having made the diagnosis and assessed the sensitivity of the organism, specific antibiotics are administered systemically and also locally, either into the shunt apparatus itself or by separate access to the ventricular system through a ventricular reservoir. Stark (1968) showed the effectiveness of treating staphylococcus albus infections with intraventricular cloxacillin in 5mg doses, and also of treating E.Coli infections with intraventricular ampicillin in a similar dosage. Table 8.1 provides a list of suitable antibiotics with dosages for intraventricular injection.

The patient should not only be clinically controlled by this treatment but the CSF and blood stream should be shown to be sterile before the next stage is undertaken. It has been generally found that the infected shunt has to be removed before permanent control of the situation can be achieved. The removal of the shunt can be followed by a period of continued treatment and control of the hydrocephalus by intermittent aspiration through a separate ventriculostomy indwelling reservoir, or, the infected shunt can be replaced immediately by a new shunt in one operative manoeuvre. The latter procedure seems more risky but has been satisfactory in the experience of various authors (Luthardt 1970, Nicholas *et al.* 1970).

TABLE 8.1
Intraventricular antibiotics
(Single daily doses suitable for infants with hydrocephalus
and infected shunts)

Name	Dosage
Ampicillin	20-50 mg
Carbenicillin	25 mg
Cephalothin	25 mg
Cephloridine	5-50 mg
Cloxacillin	5-20 mg
Colymycin (Colistimethate)	5-15 mg
Gentamycin	1-5 mg
Kanamycin	20 mg
Methicillin	50 mg
Penicillin	10-20,000 units
Polymyxin B	3-5 mg
Streptomycin	20-100 mg

Spontaneous arrest of hydrocephalus

This is a condition which occurs gradually. Its clinical manifestation is that of a child making satisfactory neurological progress with a skull circumference within the normal range but a shunt which is apparently not working when judged by palpation of the reservoir; furthermore, the time lapse since insertion of the shunt makes the likelihood of walling off of the lower end very considerable. It is assumed in these circumstances that the balance between CSF production and absorption is achieved by trans-ependymal passage of the CSF or a spontaneous fistula from the ventricular system to the subarachnoid space. The arrest is sufficiently unstable for there to be no hurry in removing the shunt apparatus and it is usually left in place until the child is beyond five years of age. Confirmation of the situation may be obtained by isotope ventriculography which shows not only that there is no passage of the isotope through the shunt system but also that the isotope is able to leave the ventricular system at a satisfactory rate, and prolonged pressure readings show a level below 10mm of mercury. The shunt is then temporarily clipped off and the child observed for three days, and if there are no untoward sequelae the shunt is finally removed (Holtzer and De Lange 1973).

CHAPTER 9

General Orthopaedic Management and Operative Treatment

W. J. W. Sharrard

Aims of Treatment

The aims of orthopaedic management are:

(1) to correct deformity, to maintain its correction, to prevent recurrence, and to avoid production of other deformities;

(2) to obtain the best possible locomotor function;

(3) to prevent or minimise the effects of sensory and motor deficiency.

These aims can only be achieved by adequate assessment of the deformity and the paralysis and by the correct use of conservative and operative treatment during infancy and childhood.

Times of Assessment

Orthopaedic assessment should be made as soon as possible after birth, preferably before closure of the spinal lesion but, if not, within two or three weeks of birth. Subsequent orthopaedic assessments should be made at least once every three months for the first year of life and once every six months thereafter until growth is complete at the age of fifteen or sixteen years. Reassessment may need to be made at any time immediately preceding an orthopaedic or neurosurgical intervention, or when there is evidence suggesting increasing deformity or alteration in the paralytic state. In addition to clinical descriptions, clinical photographs form an ideal record of deformity and its correction.

Factors in the Causation of Deformity

The factors responsible for deformity in spina bifida are:

(1) unbalanced muscle action;

(2) the effects of posture, gravity and external forces;

(3) fractures or abnormal growth of bone;

(4) co-existent congenital malformation.

The commonest cause of deformity in spina bifida is unbalanced muscle activity, whether before or after birth (Sharrard 1962). Deformity is progressive because increasing deformity results in increased mechanical advantage for the deforming muscle and mechanical disadvantage for its weak opponent. Deformity develops more rapidly in infancy and earlier childhood, probably in association with more rapid growth. It first affects muscles and tendons and then ligaments and soft tissues. Deformity at bone develops after many months, usually after the deformity has passed the extremes of range of the joints concerned (Sharrard 1973).

Deformity develops when the active but unopposed muscle does not grow as rapidly as the bone because of the lack of stimulus of its opponent (Sharrard 1967).

The paralysed muscles on the opposite side of the deformity become passively lengthened, but paralysed muscles on the same side as the deformity will shorten; for example, if tibialis anterior is acting alone in the foot it produces a calcaneo-varus deformity in which the paralysed peroneal muscles become lengthened and the paralysed tibialis posterior become shortened.

Deformities which develop early in intra-uterine life affect all of the limb structures, including the skin, and are therefore very rigid (see Chapter 3).

Deformity due to muscle imbalance is obvious in children in whom there is a clearly-defined lower motor neurone loss in certain spinal segments, with voluntary or involuntary pull of muscles opposing them. Typical patterns of paralytic deformity corresponding to the neurological deficit may be present at birth or may develop later. When they develop *in utero*, the degree of deformity may be exaggerated by additional factors such as intra-uterine posture and pressure (Ráliš 1970).

Deformity in association with upper motor neurone lesions is less likely to be present at birth since it is rare for spasticity to be exhibited *in utero*. Deformities characteristic of spastic paralysis such as flexion of the hip, flexion of the knee and equinus at the ankle may develop as a result either of a spina bifida lesion (*e.g.* myeloschisis) proximal to the lumbosacral segments, or in association with cerebral lesions or hydrocephalus.

In some patients, complex deformity may result from a combination of upper and lower motor neurone lesions or from deformity produced by intra-uterine muscle activity which has become modified after birth.

Deformities due to muscle imbalance and associated with continued activity in the deforming muscles are not amenable to correction by passive manipulation or splintage. If such measures do produce some correction of the deformity, it invariably recurs when the splintage is removed.

Deformity due to posture or to the effects of gravity is usually seen in flail joints. In rare cases it may develop *in utero*, when there is complete lower motor neurone paralysis of all muscles associated with the joint and the limb shows deformity dependent entirely on the position taken up by the infant *in utero*. More often, deformity develops after birth in joints which were not previously deformed but which have become flail. The characteristic deformities are: flexion, abduction and lateral rotation at the hips; semiflexion at the knees; and equinus of the feet. The deformities are associated with fibrosis in the tendon sheaths and joint capsules and are a secondary consequence of oedema and deposition of fibrin. Muscle and tendon shortening and joint deformity only follow at a much later time. Such deformities are amenable to repeated passive movements or to the use of splints.

Deformity in older children may be due to undetected fractures or epiphyseal displacement. Fractures of the shaft of the femur may unite with lateral rotation and flexion deformity; supracondylar fractures with epiphyseal separation tend to unite with valgus deformity at the knee; and supramalleolar fractures or fracture separations of the lower end of the tibia tend to deform into equinovarus.

A few limb deformities may be due to co-existent congenital anomalies such as hemihypertrophy, absence of the fibula, brachydactylia, absence of the foot, and occasionally metatarsus varus or talipes equinovarus, although the last is much more frequently a paralytic deformity. Deformities of the spine, apart from the spina bifida lesion itself, occur commonly, often at a different level from the main spinal defect. Hemivertebrae (sometimes multiple), variable deformities of the vertebral bodies and their associated ribs, localised or generalised kyphosis (particularly in the lumbar spine), and absence of the sacrum or of the sacrum and one or more of the lumbar vertebrae are not infrequently seen in association with spina bifida.

Special mention needs to be made of recurrent deformity. If a deformity has been corrected operatively in a part of the limb that appears to be completely paralysed *e.g.* equinus deformity at the ankle in which the tendo calcaneus has been divided with good correction, then recurrence of the deformity in spite of maintenance of passive movements of the joint should give rise to strong suspicion that there may be autonomous or semi-reflex activity in the muscle which is immune to detection by clinical means. In such an instance, electrical stimulation will often reveal activity in the muscle responsible for the recurrent deformity. In other instances, a deformity such as calcaneovarus may have been corrected and muscle balance altered by tendon transplantation but there then later follows a different deformity such as equino-valgus. In such an instance, there may have been a mixture of normal and reflex activity that has given a misleading assessment at the time of the original correction and tendon transplantation.

MOTOR ACTIVITY

The types of motor activity that may present in relation to various types of lesion of the spinal cord have been considered in earlier chapters, and methods of assessment by clinical examination and electrodiagnosis at birth, in infancy, and in later childhood have also been considered (see Chapters 4 and 6).

Detailed clinical and electrical investigation of muscle activity needs to be made before the programme of orthopaedic management is prepared: the importance of response to electrical stimulus cannot be over-emphasised. A limb that appears to be completely paralysed (particularly at the foot and ankle) may possess active muscles with lower motor neurone innervation unresponsive to voluntary control but neverthe-less capable of producing deformity and requiring orthopaedic action to balance any unbalanced activity that may be present.

One should be able to grade the strength of muscles that are under voluntary control in accordance with the M.R.C. (Medical Research Council) scale, at least when the child is old enough to be able to respond to requests to move the limb; before this time, however, it is usually only possible to record muscle activity as 'absent', 'weak', 'moderate', or 'strong'. Muscles that are not under voluntary control are more difficult to grade, although the extent of their response to electrical stimulation of given intensity may give some indication of their power.

It is convenient to record muscle activity on a muscle chart in which the muscles are listed in order of their root innervation, since this will often indicate the extent of the spinal cord and root lesion.

Patterns of Paralysis and Deformity

Certain specific lesions of the spinal cord may give rise to characteristic patterns of deformity, either at birth or developing in the course of early childhood. When there is normal innervation down to a specific neural segment with complete flaccid paralysis below this level, the pattern of deformity corresponds well with the expected imbalance of muscle activity (Sharrard 1964a, Stark and Baker 1967).

(1) Paralysis below the twelfth thoracic root

Complete paralysis in the lumbar and sacral segments results in no muscle imbalance in the lower limbs. The hips lie in slight lateral rotation, the knees in a little flexion, and the feet in slight equinus, all the elements of the posture being due to gravity alone. Progressive deformity does not develop provided that passive joint movement is maintained.

(2) Paralysis below the first lumbar root (Fig. 9.1)

There is weak flexor power at the hip due to action in the iliopsoas and sartorius muscles. The limb lies in flexion, with some abduction and lateral rotation at the hip, some flexion at the knee, and slight equinus of the foot. In time, the deformity may increase to the point where the limbs lie in right-angled abduction and right-angled flexion at the knees. The appearances may exactly simulate those of reflex sacral innervation (see below). However, the position of the hip differs in the two lesions. When there is innervation from the first lumbar root only, there is flexion and some lateral rotation deformity at the hip. The abducted hips can be adducted to the neutral so that the knees come together to reveal that the deformity is almost entirely one of flexion at the hip. This may be quite severe in a neglected child, the flexion deformity having been masked by a compensatory lumbar lordosis.

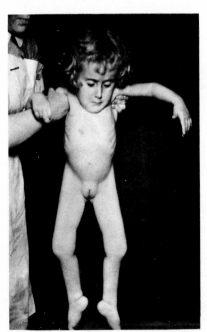

Fig. 9.1. Lower limb posture and deformity in paralysis below the third lumbar root. There is flexion, abduction and lateral rotation at the hips, some flexion at the knees, and mobile equinus of the feet.

(3) Paralysis below the second lumbar root

There is strong activity in the hip flexors, lateral rotators and adductors. There is fixed flexion at the hip, some limitation of abduction and fixed lateral rotation. The hips may be subluxated at birth and are likely to become dislocated within the first two years of life.

(4) Paralysis below the third lumbar root

There is strong power in the hip flexors and adductors and good power in the quadriceps muscle. There is considerable fixed flexion, lateral rotation and adduction deformity at the hips, which are likely to be dislocated at birth or to become dislocated during the first six months of life. There is limited flexion at the knee.

(5) Paralysis below the fourth lumbar root (Fig. 9.2)

There is normal activity in the hip flexors and adductors and in the quadriceps. Severe deformity in flexion, lateral rotation and adduction occurs at the hip and they are almost always dislocated at birth. The knee may show fixed recurvatum deformity. At the foot, there is likely to be calcaneo-varus deformity due to isolated action of the tibialis anterior.

(6) Paralysis below the fifth lumbar root (Figs. 9.3 and 6.4)

In addition to the muscles recorded above, there is activity in the gluteal abductors, the knee flexors, the tibialis posterior and the extensors of the toes. Some flexion and adduction deformity may be present at the hips, but the hip is not dislocated at birth. It may become dislocated within the first three years of life. Deformity at the knee is negligible but a calcaneus deformity develops at the foot.

(7) Paralysis below the first sacral root (Fig. 9.4)

There is little or no deformity at the hip in the early years of life, though some flexion deformity may develop in later childhood because of persistent weakness of hip extension. There is no deformity at the knee but there is often marked deformity at the foot, with paralysis of the intrinsic muscles and of the long toe flexor muscles; in some instances this may result in congenital paralytic vertical talus deformity.

(8) Paralysis below the second sacral segment (Fig. 9.5)

The only weakness is in the intrinsic muscles of the feet. There may be cavus and claw-toe deformity at birth which is likely to increase during childhood.

(9) Sacral reflex deformity (Fig. 9.6)

This is a characteristic deformity that may develop in early childhood, especially in association with a thoraco-lumbar lesion in which there is complete paralysis of all voluntary activity except in the hip flexors and with reflex activity in the sacrally-innervated muscles only. The hip adductors, the quadriceps, and all the dorsiflexors of the ankle and toes are paralysed. The hips lie in flexion, lateral rotation and abduction, and the abduction deformity is a fixed deformity so that the knees cannot be brought to meet each other in the mid line. There is severe flexion deformity of the knees and severe equinus deformity of both feet.

(10) Mixed neurological lesion

An almost infinite variety of deformities may result from various combinations of spinal cord abnormality, especially when secondary infection or degeneration has occurred in the spinal lesion. A common appearance is one in which there is a pot-hook deformity of the foot with calcaneo-valgus deformity of the hind-foot, cavus of the mid-foot and clawing of the toes or intrinsic deformity of the toes.

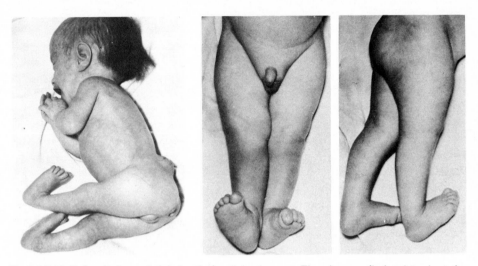

Fig. 9.2 (*left*). Deformity in paralysis below the fourth lumbar root. There is severe flexion, lateral rotation and adduction deformity at the hips, a recurvatum deformity at the knees and calcaneo-varus deformities of the feet.

Fig. 9.3 (*middle and right*). Deformity and paralysis below the fifth lumbar root. There is flexion and adduction deformity at the hips and calcaneus deformities of the feet.

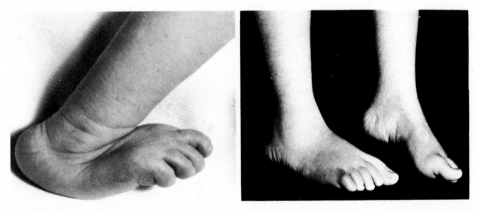

Fig. 9.4 (*left*). Congenital paralytic vertical talus deformity in paralysis below the first sacral root. The fore-foot is in calcaneo-valgus and the hind-foot in equino-valgus, with dislocation of the talo-navicular joint.

Fig. 9.5 (*right*). Cavus and claw-toe deformity in the left foot in which there is paralysis below the second sacral segment.

89

(11) Isolated root paralysis (Fig. 9.7)

In occult varieties of spina bifida or in lesions associated with lipomata of the cauda equina, there may be paralysis and deformity associated with paralysis of a single root, with activity in other roots being normal. If, for example, there is paralysis in the fifth lumbar root only, equino-varus deformity of the foot may be the only deformity present.

Deformity in the trunk is less often attributable to paralytic imbalance, though paralysis of the lower thoracic roots may give rise to abdominal weakness and secondary lordotic deformity, especially in late childhood and adolescence. More often, deformity in the spine arises as a result of abnormal bone growth. Single or multiple hemivertebra formation is usually associated with congenital scoliosis which is liable to increase and to become a severe deformity in later childhood. Spina bifida in which the vertebral bodies are normal is not necessarily associated with any deformity during the early years of life, but scoliosis may gradually develop and then become a severe lordoscoliosis after the age of ten, when rapid growth of the vertebral bodies occurs. With it can develop pelvic obliquity, and this, together with hip deformity associated with paralysis (as described above) may produce a complex situation in which a child previously able to walk to a limited extent becomes unable to do so.

Kyphotic deformity of the lumbar spine is likely to be associated with severe open spina bifida deformity of the spine (Hoppenfeld 1967), and, when present and obvious at birth, is almost always associated with severe neurological deficit. Lesser degrees of kyphosis may, however, be present without such an extensive neurological defect, but a laterally placed erector spinae mass may fail to act as an extensor of the lumbar spine or may become perverted into a flexor with development of increasing kyphotic deformity during childhood (Drennan 1970). Increasing kyphotic deformity may then lead to secondary increase in lower limb paralysis (see Chapter 3).

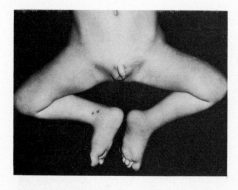

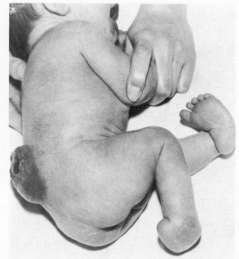

Fig. 9.6 *(above)*. Sacral reflex deformity. There is flexion-abduction deformity at the hips, severe flexion deformity at the knees and equinus deformity at the feet.

Fig. 9.7 *(right)*. Equinovarus deformity of the feet due to isolated paralysis of the fifth lumbar root.

SENSORY FUNCTION

Accurate assessment of sensory loss cannot be made until the child is at least six years old. In the newborn, crying in response to pin-prick or skin stimulation during electrical testing may give a rough estimate of the sensory level (see Chapter 6), and tickling or pinching the skin in infants and young children may produce an appropriate general response. Movement of the limb (in response to stimulation of skin) unaccompanied by a general arousal of the child is more likely to be a reflex response than a voluntary action and its main value is in establishing that there is an intact sensory axon.

When sensibility can be more accurately assessed, it is often found that the areas of normal sensory supply correspond with the level of motor innervation, but this is by no means constant. It is always advisable to assume that areas supplied by the sacral neural segments (particularly the perineum and the feet) are insensitive and therefore liable to pressure ulceration. Assessment of sensory function by the measurement of evoked responses is of limited value; when there is a positive response, the presence of some sensibility can be assumed, but a negative response may be due to the presence of hydrocephalus.

Vasomotor function in spina bifida has been the subject of very little investigation (Porter 1968). In general, completely flail lower limbs associated with complete loss of motor and sensory nerve roots show vasomotor paralysis with cyanosis, a liability to chilblains, and oedema. The presence of intact sensory nerves, even when there is no general sensory arousal because of the spinal cord lesion, seems to prevent gross vasomotor changes in the skin and normal skin sweating may be present.

Lack of proprioception of the superficial and deep structures in the lower limbs is one of the factors that may result in lack of co-ordination and balance in efforts to walk in childhood. That this is not the only factor is illustrated by the finding that children with congenital hydrocephalus often show delay in walking and difficulties in balance probably due to poor spatial orientation and cerebellar deficiencies. These factors may delay the establishment of walking (even with aids) beyond the age of four years in children who otherwise would seem to have satisfactory lower limb musculature.

The Management of Lower Limb Paralysis and Deformity
General Aims of Orthopaedic Management

In order to achieve the combined aims of correction of deformity and improvement of function in a child suffering from a disease with multiple handicaps, certain conditions have to be observed.

Before a programme of orthopaedic treatment is planned, an adequate assessment of the paralysis and deformity must be made. At the same time, the general condition of the child, the presence of any hydrocephalus, the adequacy of any measures needed to control it, and the adequacy of renal function must be taken into consideration. Orthopaedic treatment must be integrated with other specialist treatment; in general, measures relating to the neurological and urological problems must take priority over orthopaedic measures (Menelaus 1971a).

Where there is deformity at several joints (or possibly at all joints) in the lower limbs, a programme of orthopaedic management will need to be planned. With regard to the extent of the paralysis in the limbs, it should be possible, within reasonable limits, to assess the ultimate goal of treatment, *i.e.,* walking without aids, walking with calipers of varying extent, limited walking combined with a wheelchair existence or complete wheelchair existence. Decisions can then be made about correction of deformity. The aim should be to correct deformities in sequence until the limbs sufficiently approach the normal to allow walking or the fitting of calipers which will enable the child to learn to walk. In contrast with the management of congenital deformity without spina bifida, it is seldom appropriate to commence active treatment at birth. The requirements of the neurosurgical management of the spinal lesion and any hydrocephalus take priority and it may not be appropriate to perform surgical, manipulative or plaster treatment in the newborn period. Apart from assessment of paralysis and deformity, orthopaedic management in the first weeks is confined to the maintenance of passive movements of the joints of the lower limbs. It is possible to obtain some correction of foot deformity in the neonatal period by carefully applied elastic strapping in infants with extensive paralysis of muscles below the knee (Walker 1971). Active measures to correct deformity are usually begun at about six months of life and continue during the first two years, the aim being to correct deformity so as to allow the fitting of calipers and the development of walking ability between the second and the fourth year; in some instances, complications arising in other systems will interrupt orthopaedic treatment and may extend or delay correction until after the age of six months.

Basic principles of orthopaedic management
The same basic principles apply to any individual joint in the lower limbs:—
(1) Conservative correction is contra-indicated in most deformities because of the liability to produce sores in anaesthetic skin and because of the liability to osteoporosis and fractures in limbs immobilised for long periods. Since muscle imbalance is the predominant cause of deformity in spina bifida, conservative measures are unlikely to be successful.
(2) Deformity should be corrected by elongation of short tendons, muscles and associated soft tissues. Provided this is done before the age of three or four years, it is often possible to correct even severe deformities without resort to operations upon bone.
(3) Muscle activity should be balanced by tendon transfer, by partial or total muscle denervation, or by tendon or muscle excision. Ideally, muscle balancing operations should be performed at the same time as tendon and soft-tissue lengthening, or shortly after.
(4) Immobilisation after operation should continue for the minimum time necessary to allow healing of the soft tissues and sound re-attachment of transplanted muscles. This need rarely last longer than four weeks.
(5) If deformity remains after maximum correction of soft tissues has been made, further correction should be obtained by bony correction such as osteotomy or excision of bone and cartilage, even in young children. Failure to correct

deformity as completely as possible, especially in the foot, is likely to lead to serious secondary consequences of ulceration and infection when weight is put on the limb.

(6) After removal of plaster fixation, persistent use of splinting (except that required to allow walking) is inadvisable, partly because it discourages active use of muscles, including transplanted muscles, and also because it leads to increased osteoporosis and liability to spontaneous fractures.

(7) When deformity has been corrected at all joints, one can begin a planned programme to promote the ability to walk with the aid of suitable appliances. The programme will involve braces, supports and physiotherapy.

The Place of Operative Surgery

Operative treatment can be used in three ways: (1) to correct deformity, (2) to modify muscle activity, or (3) to stabilise weak or flail joints.

Correction of deformity

(1) *Tendon surgery.* Since relative shortness of tendons is the commonest factor in the production of deformity in spina bifida, correction of tendon length is the commonest feature of operations to correct deformity. Almost any muscle having sufficient length of tendon can be elongated by a *Z* technique. Tendon elongation is usually accompanied by slight diminution of about one grade in the strength of the tendon. It is indicated when continued functioning of the tendon is required.

Simple tenotomy can also be used to correct deformity and is primarily indicated when a short tendon has been shown to be functionless by clinical and electrical testing before operation. Although a single tendon may sometimes be divided subcutaneously, open tenotomy is much more often needed to ensure adequate release of all affected tendons and soft tissues. Even if a considerable gap is left after division of a tendon, there is no guarantee that the tendon will not restore its own continuity by subsequent growth; this is particularly likely to occur if the muscle has reflex activity. It seems possible that the continuing pull of the tendon stimulates further growth of the fibres. The tendo calcaneus is particularly liable to produce recurrent deformity by this means. Tenotomy, combined with excision of a substantial length of tendon, may overcome this problem in older children but even this may not be sufficient to prevent tendon regrowth in infants.

Correction of a deformity due to a short tendon is often accompanied by transplantation of that tendon; if this is done, it is important that the tendon sheath (or paratenon) should be removed, otherwise a partial regrowth of the tendon to its old insertion may occur. A common example of this is seen in transplantation of the extensor hallucis longus tendon to the first metatarsal; tendon fibres may sprout to rejoin their original insertion and even detach themselves from the transplanted site.

(2) *Fascial, ligamentous and capsular release.* After division of tendons, there is often sufficient length in other soft tissues (including capsules and ligaments of joints) to allow complete correction of deformity, especially in infancy. If not, transverse division of fascial, ligamentous and capsular structures should be made, even if this involves opening joints to achieve correction and even if, at times, some separation of

the bones concerned in the articulation occurs, as, for instance, at the ankle and subtaloid joints in release of varus deformity. The aim should always be to restore the normal range of movements at the deformed joint.

(3) *Osteotomy*. Correction of deformity by bone division, with or without removal of a wedge of bone, may be indicated when division of tendons and other soft tissues has failed to correct deformity completely or when tension on vessels or nerves prevents further correction. Some types of deformity can be corrected only by osteotomy, *e.g.* rotational deformities of the thigh or leg. Correction by osteotomy is more often needed in older children or when multiple soft tissue corrections have failed; in adolescence, correction may sometimes be combined with arthrodesis of a joint for stability.

Modification of Muscle Activity

The most common method of correcting muscle imbalance in spina bifida is by tendon transfer. Decisions as to which tendon should be transferred and the site to which it should be inserted must depend greatly on assessment of muscle activity before operation. Ideally, a transferred tendon will achieve its best function when its new action bears some relation to its previous action, *e.g.* when a dorsiflexor tendon of the ankle or foot is transferred medially or laterally and still remains a dorsiflexor. However, when a tendon is a major factor in the production of the deformity, it is all right to transfer this tendon so that it works in the direction opposite to that in which it worked before. It may not be possible to demonstrate voluntary activity in the transferred tendon but it may nevertheless act strongly to prevent recurrence of deformity. The transplantation, for example, of two of the dorsiflexor tendons through the interosseous membrane to the tendo calcaneus will prevent the recurrence of calcaneus deformity even though relatively little active plantar flexion can be demonstrated after operation. That such a mechanism is important is demonstrated by the fact that when there is only a single strong muscle acting on a joint, the transfer of that tendon to a new site may produce a new deformity. If, for example, the tibialis anterior is the only muscle acting below the knee and it is transferred through the interosseous membrane into the tendo calcaneus, it can produce equinus deformity.

In the ideal situation the transfer of appropriate tendons produces an even balance of muscle activity in a joint, and this can be very satisfactory both for function and for the prevention of further deformity. Difficulties may arise when it is not possible to assess accurately the function of muscles before operation, and this is found particularly in limbs with extensive reflex or autonomous muscle activity. If there is doubt, it is better to perform a simple elongation, or, to transfer only a single tendon and await the results of this operation before deciding on any further tendon transfers. Occasionally, due to severe deformity, a tendon may be too short to reach to its new insertion. If so, it may be necessary to elongate the tendon at one procedure and to transfer it four to six weeks later, when the new lengthened tendon has reformed.

Partial or total denervation of a muscle may sometimes be the only means by which muscle imbalance can be corrected. Such is the situation when there is excessive action in the intrinsic muscles of the feet which requires selective plantar denervation of muscles causing deformity (Garceau and Brahms 1956). An alternative solution occasionally needed is complete excision of a muscle and its tendon, a solution that may be indicated when more than two unsuccessful attempts have been made to correct muscle imbalance due to predominant activity in a single muscle or muscle group.

Stabilisation of Joints

Stabilisation of joints by arthrodesis is likely to be indicated in children over the age of twelve, usually at the ankle or foot. Until this age, stabilisation may have been achieved by the use of braces or calipers; arthrodesis operations are indicated to allow these apparatuses to be discarded. It is often possible, at the same time, to correct any remaining elements of deformity by appropriate excision of bone.

Arthrodesis in younger children may occasionally be indicated in special circumstances. Examples are (a) extra-articular subtaloid fusion (Grice 1952) for a flail foot that tends to go into valgus and cannot be held by suitable footwear and bracing or (b) calcaneo-cuboid arthrodesis in varus of the forefoot when it is intended to diminish growth in the outer side of the foot. In a similar way, fusion of the joints on one side of the spine may be indicated in young children to diminish excessive growth on that side of the spine in the presence of a hemivertebra.

The Timing of Surgical Procedures

The age of the patient should be no bar to the performance of corrective surgery, and progressive deformity is an absolute indication for surgery whatever the age. Certain qualifications in relation to age are relevant. Surgery on the limbs below the age of six months is inadvisable in most instances because of the more important requirements of neurosurgery and general management. Accurate assessment of muscle activity is difficult in very young children and the pattern of muscle activity may not become stable until after six months. The small size of structures, especially in the foot, makes operations such as tendon transfer difficult at this age, and operative treatment should normally be confined to simple tenotomies or tendon elongations, if these are absolutely necessary.

The ideal time for correction of many deformities of any part of the limb is between the sixth month and second year of life. Correction of tendon length combined with appropriate muscle-balancing procedures is often sufficient to allow complete correction of deformities that at first sight seem unpromising. If a deformity recurs, a second or even a third operation may sometimes be needed, the aim being to correct all deformity by the time the child is two or three years old so that appropriate bracing and instruction in walking can begin.

Between the ages of two and five years, correction of tendon length and release of soft tissues may not be sufficient to produce satisfactory correction of deformity and the addition of osteotomy is more often needed. During this period, the deformity that has not been corrected completely at an earlier time or the deformity that has recurred may need further surgery. Sometimes, the general condition of the child has made it impossible to proceed with orthopaedic surgical treatment at an earlier age.

95

In all but a few patients, however, the aim should be to obtain the best correction possible by the time the child is five years old and about to start its education.

Between the ages of five and twelve years, surgery should be needed only for those infants who have developed a recurrent deformity which was not present previously but which is increasing and causing problems in the fitting of braces or is facilitating the development of pressure sores.

After twelve years, the final corrective surgery (particularly surgery upon bones) may be needed, either to correct deformities of the spine or to stabilise joints of the foot.

Contra-indications to Surgery of the Limbs

The only absolute contra-indication to surgery at any particular time is an inadequate general state of health of the child, as indicated by severe renal dysfunction or severe cerebral dysfunction. Consideration may also have to be given to the extent of the procedures that may be advised or the number of such procedures. A child with poor renal function may be fit enough to allow one or two minor procedures to be performed to make satisfactory management and nursing possible or to prevent incipient sores but may not be fit enough to undergo surgery to produce complete correction at all joints.

Intellectual impairment, by itself, is not a contra-indication to orthopaedic procedures. An intellectual quotient as low as 50 is not necessarily incompatible with ability to gain some independent walking function, and, provided the child's general health is adequate, such a child should not be denied the benefit orthopaedic surgery can give in helping him to achieve his maximum potential function.

THE PLACE OF CONSERVATIVE MEASURES— PHYSIOTHERAPY, SPLINTAGE AND BRACING

Physiotherapy

Physiotherapy has a very important part to play for the child with spina bifida (Martin 1964, 1967), particularly in teaching and training in stance, walking and independent activities. The physiotherapist forms an important link between the parent and the surgical and medical teams and is well placed to assess the detailed problems that are likely to arise for a child and for the parents. It is important that the physiotherapist should recognise the limitation of physiotherapeutic treat-ment and, particularly for those who have been accustomed to treat children with cerebral palsy or poliomyelitis, there must be an appreciation of the specific problems that may arise from anaesthetic skin and bone fragility.

In the over-all assessment of disability and function, a physiotherapist often has particular opportunities to discover specific defects and difficulties which the surgeon or paediatrician may not be able to discover in the course of routine examination. Most physiotherapists can contribute a great deal of useful informa-tion about individual muscle activity and can appreciate the development of progressive deformity or difficulties arising in bracing that may not be apparent during normal clinical examination.

Prevention of deformity

The physiotherapist must appreciate that there is very little that can be done by physiotherapeutic means to correct a rigid deformity or to prevent progressive deformity due to muscle imbalance. Deformity due to habitual posture can be minimised or prevented by daily passive movement, and instructions in the performance of such passive movements can be given to most parents.

Management after surgery

As soon as plaster fixation has been removed, the physiotherapist can help to mobilise stiff joints by the gentle use of passive movements and exercises. There must be an awareness of the fragility of bone following a period of immobilisation in plaster and recognition of the fact that swelling of a limb in such circumstances is almost always indicative of the development of a fracture or epiphyseal separation.

Encouragement of movement in muscles that are active or in muscles that have been transplanted is the most important measure that the physiotherapist can apply, and a knowledge of the ways in which such activity may be produced in infants and young children is essential.

Walking training

The achievement of independent walking is the ultimate goal for any child with spina bifida. Provided that severe cerebral complications have not occurred and orthopaedic measures have succeeded in correcting deformity and producing balanced muscle activity, a high proportion of children with spina bifida should become capable of some kind of independent walking, even those with complete lower limb paralysis.

Due to the difficulties, effort and extensive bracing involved in walking only short distances, some children, on reaching adolescence, may discard the limited ability for walking that they have acquired in favour of a complete wheel-chair existence (Hoffer *et al.* 1973). However, this possibility should not deter the physiotherapist from attempting to gain as much independent function as can be inspired in a young child.

(Rehabilitation and methods of walking training will be discussed in a later section.)

Splintage

The place of splintage in the management of paralysis and deformity in spina bifida is the subject of some confusion and dispute. Confusion has arisen because conditions such as congenital dislocation of the hip and talipes equinovarus in otherwise normal children are treated successfully by appropriate splintage. Splintage also plays an important part in the prevention of deformity in early poliomyelitis and in the management of a number of orthopaedic conditions in childhood. It is difficult, therefore, to appreciate that splintage of a similar type does not necessarily achieve the same results with spina bifida patients, and, in some circumstances, may even have a detrimental effect.

An important factor that limits the use of splintage in the correction of deformity in spina bifida is the presence of anaesthesia in areas of skin that are subject to pressure. Whereas a normal child would respond to excessive pressure on the skin by crying (in infancy) or complaining (in childhood), the spina bifida child will tolerate excessive pressure without symptoms or complaint, with serious results. Even if splints or plaster casts are applied without excessive pressure and with adequate padding, sores may result from movements caused by unbalanced muscle activity inside the plaster or splints and these may cause ulceration.

Although it is not easy to conceive that deformity due to unbalanced muscle activity can progress when a rigid splint has been applied to the limb, there is now irrefutable evidence that in any paralytic condition in which there is unbalanced muscle activity, deformity will progress in a growing child in spite of all conservative measures (Sharrard 1967). Splintage can prevent deformity due solely to posture or the effects of gravity in a limb in which there is either complete paralysis or in which muscle activity is balanced. It is equally true that a splint can produce deformity by imposing a fixed posture on the limb in the absence of any muscle activity capable of correcting it. For example, in a child suffering from paralytic dislocation of the hips with activity only in the hip flexors and adductors, release of the adductors and splintage of the hips in flexion and *abduction* will produce a fixed deformity in flexion and abduction. When the splint is removed (although the hips may be reduced satisfactorily), the iliopsoas and other flexors become perverted abductors and maintain the hip in the former splinted position indefinitely, since there are no hip extensors and medial rotators to restore the normal position of the lower limbs.

For all these reasons, splints in children with spina bifida should be used sparingly and appropriately. At the hips, splintage in abduction to limit progress towards dislocation in an infant or child with weak hip abductors is a useful measure but the splint must hold the hips in abduction, medial rotation and extension, not in abduction, lateral rotation and flexion (McKibbin 1973). Such a splint may have considerable virtue in preventing dislocation until good assessment can be made of the activity of the hip musculature and appropriate tendon transfers or until other surgical measures can be applied.

In the infant, progressive plaster casts can be used with care to correct deformity such as equinus or equinovarus, provided that there is no excessive muscle imbalance. The best results are achieved when there is complete paralysis below the knee and the deformity is essentially due to intra-uterine posture or pressure. Once correction has been achieved it is doubtful whether continued splintage is necessary, since daily passive movements are likely to maintain correction of deformity in an ankle and foot that is completely flail. Similarly, at the knee, flexion deformity may arise in a flail limb which tends to fall into flexion and abduction at the hips and flexion at the knees; a simple plastic splint may prevent or minimise deformity if simple passive movements prove inadequate, but such a splint will fail if there is strong activity (especially if it is also spastic) in the hamstring muscles in the presence of a weak or paralysed quadriceps muscle.

The use of night splints is the subject of some dispute. If carefully fitted and appropriately applied, night splints can maintain the correct posture of a limb, but, at the same time, there is considerable danger of producing pressure sores if the splint becomes displaced during the night, or if it becomes too small or is applied incorrectly. On the whole, the dangers of ulceration due to night splintage probably outweigh the benefits of their use. The author's experience shows that when night splints have been completely discarded the incidence of deformity is no greater than in patients who regularly used night splints.

When splintage is used, it should always be discarded for some portion of the day. This allows free action of the limbs so that such muscle activity as is present will be encouraged; also, the liability to progressive osteoporosis of the lower limb bones by prolonged immobility is thus minimised.

Bracing

The essential function of bracing is to give support to weak joints and so make it possible for the patient to stand and walk. The same limitations that apply to splintage in relation to deformity apply to the use of braces.

Most classical and conventional forms of bracing are essentially a form of exo-skeleton applied in such a way as to limit and stabilise the unwanted joint movements that are the subject of absent or inadequate muscle control.

Depending on the degree of paralysis, bracing may be needed in the form of below-knee irons or double irons for an unstable foot and ankle, a full caliper for an unstable knee, a full caliper with pelvic band for an unstable hip, and a full caliper with trunk support for an unstable lower trunk and hip. In general, it is inappropriate to apply braces until a child is judged capable of bearing weight and commencing training in walking. There may sometimes be virtue in applying bracing to allow the patient to become used to being upright, even though he may not yet have gained sufficient neurological maturity to comprehend the basic necessities for locomotion. Even then, such braces must be applied with care to those who are hydrocephalic, in whom problems of vertigo make them very frightened of being upright until they have become gradually accustomed to it.

The simplest and lightest types of brace should be used for children below the age of four years. Hinges at hip level can be introduced at the age of three or four years and knee hinges at the age of five so that the child can flex his knees while sitting at a desk at school.

Braces need to be very carefully fitted and applied in spina bifida children, much more so than in other children with paralytic lesions. Mal-alignment of a brace can easily give rise to a pressure sore and attempts to fit a brace to a child with fixed deformity at the ankle, knee or hip can sometimes be disastrous. Ideally, bracing should be delayed until any significant fixed deformity has been corrected surgically. The greatest difficulties in the application of bracing arise in children with scoliosis associated with pelvic obliquity, in those with unilateral dislocation of the hip, or those with fixed flexion or adduction deformities at one or both hips. In some patients, it may be possible, with considerable orthotic expertise, to fit a child with such a brace in spite of the deformity; the deformity will nevertheless progress inside the splint, and the splint may mask the degree of deformity and disability that is occurring. Braces also need to be inspected regularly to make sure that they are still of the correct length and dimensions; most types of brace have means built in to allow elongation of the brace to accommodate growth.

Several different types of brace have been designed specifically for the use of children with spina bifida associated with severe lower limb paralysis. Consideration of these appliances will be made in a later section devoted to walking training.

Footwear is a very important consideration in children with spina bifida because of their liability to deformities of the feet. The feet of these children are often insensitive and liable to pressure sores. Boots and shoes need to be made of soft material able to yield to minor deformity, laced open to the toe so that the foot can be put into it without curling of the toes. Where some degree of deformity has to be accepted, the use of moulded insoles helps to distribute the pressure of weight bearing. In children with spina bifida, the foot is as likely to be in calcaneus as it is to be in equinus; particular attention needs to be paid to the possibility of excessive pressure being applied to the heel. Circulatory problems in the feet and a liability to chilblains can be managed by the use of boots lined with lambswool for insulation (Menelaus 1971a).

The control of excessive passive mobility towards calcaneus requires the provision of front stops to the heel socket for a caliper, just as a flail foot tending towards equinus needs back stops or possibly stops in both directions. Inside T straps to help control passive valgus deformity or outside T straps to control passive varus deformity may be appropriate. Particular attention sometimes needs to be paid to problems of pressure on the toes and, for this reason, rigid toe caps should be avoided. Footwear specifically designed for use in spina bifida and incorporating an open front with lacing that will accommodate a variety of shapes and size of foot has some advantages.

CHAPTER 10

Specific Orthopaedic Problems

W. J. W. Sharrard

MANAGEMENT OF THE HIP

Flexion and Flexion—Lateral Rotation Deformity

Flexion deformity of more than 20 degrees requires operative correction and this can be achieved by the release of the hip flexor tendons and muscles for deformities of up to 60 degrees in a child up to the age of about 10 years. Through an oblique incision in the upper thigh, all the flexor structures that are likely to be tight can be exposed. The most important tendon to be released is the iliopsoas tendon which should be approached first. If flexion is not associated with much lateral rotation deformity, elongation of the iliopsoas tendon by a Z incision with suture of the ends and lengthening of the sartorius, tensor fasciae latae and rectus femoris as required will correct moderate or even severe flexion deformity and will weaken flexor power to a degree sufficient to prevent recurrence in most instances. In severe deformity, the iliofemoral ligaments of the hip joints may also need to be divided. If there is a marked element of lateral rotation deformity, the iliopsoas tendon may be detached from its insertion (Fig. 10.1) and transplanted beneath the femoral nerve to the anterior aspect of the greater trochanter, where it becomes a flexor and medial rotator. If fixed lateral rotation deformity is still present after the iliopsoas tendon has been divided, Menelaus (1971*a*) advises posterior exploration and division of the short lateral rotators as well.

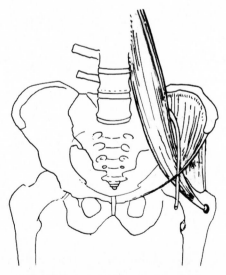

Fig. 10.1. Anterior iliopsoas transplant.

Flexion and flexion—lateral rotation deformity of more than 60 degrees may not be able to be corrected by soft tissue release alone. Further correction can be obtained after the flexor release wound has healed by an intertrochanteric extension and medial rotation osteotomy with removal of up to two cm of femoral shaft, and internal fixation with a plate and screws or a nail-plate.

Flexion-Adduction Deformity

Flexion-adduction deformity is usually associated with strong activity in the flexor and adductor muscles and weakness or complete paralysis of the gluteal muscles. Increasing fixed deformity is invariably associated with progressive sub-luxation leading to dislocation of the hip. In the most severe instances of imbalance, with innervation down to the third or fourth lumbar segment and paralysis below this level, dislocation occurs *in utero* and produces a congenital paralytic dislocation of the hip (Fig. 10.2). In instances of less severe imbalance, there may be subluxation at birth leading to dislocation between the sixth month and second year or sometimes even later. In mild cases, if no action is taken to prevent slowly increasing deformity, dislocation can occur as late as the eleventh or twelfth year of life.

(a) *Flexion-adduction deformity with dislocation at birth*

There is usually a severe fixed deformity and the hip cannot be reduced manually. The splintage normally used for congenital dislocation of the hip cannot be applied and no useful treatment can be given immediately after birth except for attempts to maintain the range of movements by gentle passive stretching. Once neurosurgical procedures have succeeded in repairing the spinal defect and con-trolling hydrocephalus, an adequate open operative adductor release, possibly with lengthening of the iliopsoas tendon, may allow the dislocation to be reduced (Fig. 10.3). Reduction can be maintained for several months by the use of splintage in abduction and medial rotation. This procedure has the merit that it encourages the development of a satisfactory acetabulum and femoral head. If adductor and flexor release is not possible during the early months of life, reduction can almost always be achieved without undue difficulty between the ninth and twelfth month of life by an adequate adductor release and open reduction of the dislocation with capsulorraphy.

Whichever of the measures described is used, the persistent paralysis of the gluteal abductors and extensors requires a further operative procedure to restore muscle balance and this can be achieved by postero-lateral iliopsoas transplantation (Sharrard 1964b). The transplant operation can be done at any age, but the ideal time is between the ninth and eighteenth month of life. Before the transplantation is made, a full range of abduction must have been obtained and if any recurrence of adduction has occurred following earlier adductor release procedures, a further adductor release may be needed. The iliopsoas muscle is transplanted through a foramen made in the wing of the ilium just lateral to the sacro-iliac joint and the tendon is attached to the postero-lateral aspect of the greater trochanter (Fig. 10.4).

Several reviews of the results of this transfer have been made (Cruess and Turner 1970, Carroll and Sharrard 1972, Freehafer *et al.* 1972, Rueda and Carroll 1972, Weisl and Matthews 1973). The capacity of the transplanted tendon to produce active abduction or extension is variable; in about 40 per cent of those in whom there is no gluteal action before operation, moderate or weak abduction can be demonstrated, but active voluntary extension is seldom found. Electromyography has shown that the transplant is active in the stance phase of walking and it seems likely that it can act as a muscular tenodesis (Buisson and Hamblen 1972). Its most important function is in the prevention of recurrence and adduction deformity and in the maintenance of reduction of the dislocation of the hip, provided that adequate reduction has been achieved at the time of operation (Fig. 10.5).

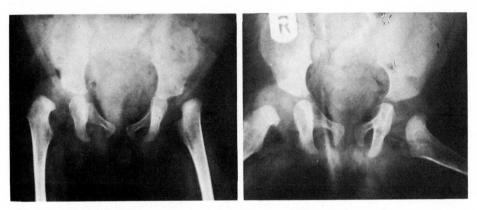

Fig. 10.2 (*left*). Radiograph of congenital paralytic dislocation of both hips.
Fig. 10.3 (*right*). Radiograph of reduction of congenital paralytic dislocation of both hips following open adductor release at age five months.

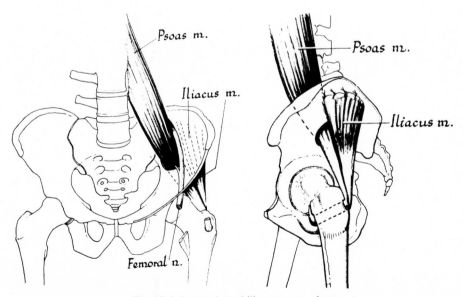

Fig. 10.4. Postero-lateral iliopsoas transplant.

103

Valgus and anteversion of the femoral neck is commonly present in congenital paralytic dislocation of the hip, but if reduction is achieved before the age of eighteen months, osteotomy to correct deformity of the femoral neck is not an automatic requirement and spontaneous correction of the bony deformity is the rule once muscle balance has been achieved.

Functional stability at the hip in walking is often sufficient to allow any bracing at hip level to be discarded, though the child may need partial brace support at hip level for several months after operative treatment has been completed. The transplant seldom acts sufficiently powerfully to prevent a Trendelenberg gait.

Sometimes a child born with bilateral congenital paralytic dislocations of the hip may, when examined at the age of six or nine months, be found to have complete flaccid or spastic paraplegia that will inevitably require the use of extensive bracing. Rueda and Carroll (1972) emphasise the futility of efforts to reduce and stabilise dislocated hips in children in this situation; operative treatment should be confined to simple tendon division and elongation or osteotomy to correct fixed deformity so that braces can be applied.

(b) *Flexion-adduction deformity with subluxation or delayed dislocation*

In this situation, there is usually some activity in the gluteal abductors. Although there is no severe deformity at birth, limited abduction and extension develops and leads to progressive subluxation and eventual dislocation. As soon as the progressive deformity is clinically and radiologically recognisable, operative treatment should be instituted to prevent further deterioration. An adequate adductor release combined with postero-lateral iliopsoas transplantation if gluteal activity is found to be weak (below grade three) gives excellent results. If clinical and electrical testing suggests that there is adequate gluteal musculature, adductor release and iliopsoas tendon lengthening alone may suffice to correct deformity and muscle imbalance.

(c) *Established dislocation in childhood*

A child four or five years old may present with an established dislocation that has either been present since birth or has developed during childhood but has not received any corrective treatment. If the muscle activity is of good quality and the child is generally healthy in other respects, the extensive procedures required to reduce dislocation and maintain it are well worthwhile, even up to the age of 10 or 11 years of age, especially if the dislocation is unilateral. In addition to deformity due to short flexor and adductor muscles, there is usually marked valgus and anteversion deformity of the femoral neck and a shallow and mal-orientated acetabulum.

Correction of the deformity can be made in one or more stages. Among the procedures required are an adequate adductor release, including the proximal hamstring origin, flexor release and postero-lateral iliopsoas transplantation, open reduction of the dislocation of the hip with capsulorraphy, innominate osteotomy of the Salter or Chiari type and varus intertrochanteric femoral osteotomy, possibly with removal of a short length of the upper end of the femur and possibly combined with extension or rotation to complete the correction of the deformity. If a late dislocation is found bilaterally, it is often better to ignore the dislocation and to concentrate on correction of deformity by adductor and flexor release, combined, if necessary, with intertrochanteric osteotomy.

Abduction—Lateral Rotation Deformity

This is a rare variety of deformity which is found when there is paralysis of all lumbar neural segments and reflex activity in isolated sacral segments. The gluteal and short lateral rotators are spastic and strong and there is associated flexion deformity of the knee due to unopposed spastic hamstring musculature.

The deformity is a difficult one to correct and requires extensive release of the gluteal musculature, either proximally or distally, or both, combined with denervation by division of the superior and inferior gluteal nerves. Even this may not be sufficient to maintain correction to allow caliper fitting, and intertrochanteric adduction-medial rotation osteotomy may be needed as well.

Gluteus Maximus Paresis

Innervation down to the first sacral segment is not associated with dislocation, and flexion deformity of any significance rarely develops, but the weakness of the gluteus maximus may produce a characteristic and ugly gait, the child tending to walk with the hips flexed and the buttocks projecting back prominently. Considerable improvement in gait (but at the expense of some weakening of flexor power at the hip) can be obtained by posterior transplantation of the iliopsoas tendon to the insertion of the gluteus maximus (see Fig. 10.6 and Sharrard 1971).

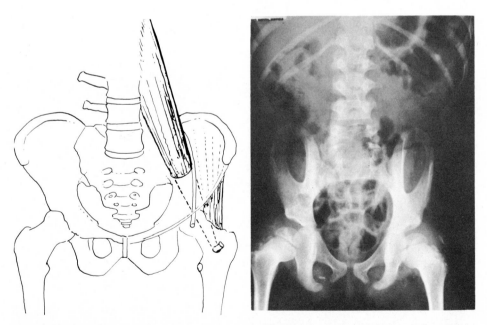

Fig. 10.5 (*left*). Maintenance of reduction of dislocated hips following postero-lateral iliopsoas transplant.
Fig. 10.6 (*right*). Posterior iliopsoas transplant.

105

MANAGEMENT OF THE KNEE

Deformity at the knee may occur in any direction—into flexion, extension (recurvatum), valgus, varus or medial or lateral rotation. In general, flexion and extension deformities are more often the result of muscle imbalance; varus and valgus deformities are due to bone deformity secondary to a spontaneous fracture or separation of the lower femoral or upper tibial epiphysis.

Flexion Deformity

Flexion deformity seldom presents as a fixed deformity at birth but is not uncommonly seen in children with a reflex pattern of innervation in which there is weakness or complete paralysis of voluntary extension by the quadriceps and spastic activity in the flexor muscles. More than 20 degrees of flexion deformity makes the fitting of calipers difficult, and if the deformity becomes much greater·than this it progresses rapidly in spite of passive movements or adequate splintage.

In mild instances, hamstring elongation or division may be sufficient to correct the deformity but if it is severe or has recurred, transplantation of two or more hamstring tendons to the lower end of the femur or to the patella may be indicated to correct muscle imbalance.

If flexion deformity is greater than 20 degrees or if division of the hamstring tendons and the posterior fascia at the knee fails to correct deformity completely, then posterior capsulectomy does not usually prove to be successful and complete correction is better achieved by supracondylar extension osteotomy of the femur with removal of a wedge of bone based anteriorly. Supracondylar extension osteotomy can also be used when flexion deformity has arisen as the result of spontaneous fracture in a flail limb. If care is taken, stability can usually be obtained without the need for internal fixation, but, in an older child, and particularly where there have been previous fractures, it may prove impossible to maintain stability and internal fixation may be needed.

Extension Deformity

Recurvatum deformity or limited knee flexion is sometimes found at birth in association with innervation down to the fourth lumbar segment and paralysis distal to this level. The quadriceps is strong and the only muscles that might flex the knee (*i.e.* the sartorius and the gracilis) prolapse anteriorly over the medial condyle of the femur and become secondary extensors of the knee.

If there is recurvatum deformity such that passive flexion of the knee is less than 20 degrees, the deformity is likely to persist unless it is corrected by operative elongation of the quadriceps (Curtis and Fisher 1969). At the same time, the sartorius and gracilis tendons can be re-attached more posteriorly on the tibia, and additional knee flexor power obtained by transplantation of the adductor magnus tendon to the semitendinosus tendon.

If the range of knee flexion is more than 40 degrees, correction by surgical elongation of the quadriceps is not generally advisable. A gradual improvement in the range of knee flexion is usually obtained as a result of spontaneous activity combined with repeated passive flexion.

Varus and Valgus Deformities

Varus and valgus deformities, which are commonly due to spontaneous fractures of the lower end of the femur or the upper end of the tibia, can be corrected by an appropriate osteotomy or by unilateral epiphyseal stapling. Occasionally, valgus deformity may be aggravated by a strong and spastic biceps femoris and a tight tensor fasciae latae, both of which may need to be divided.

MANAGEMENT OF THE FOOT

Foot deformity presents more problems than any other in spina bifida. Almost any variety of deformity may present at the ankle, hind-foot or fore-foot in equinus, calcaneus, varus, valgus, adduction or abduction. In all but the most lightly paralysed, the soles of the feet are insensitive and are liable to skin break-down over points of high pressure (Hayes and Gross 1963). With growth, the liability to pressure ulceration in the soles of the feet increases in early adolescence, when increase in size and weight of the trunk is not matched by growth of the feet (Hay and Walker 1973). A foot in which there is some mild residual deformity may be safe during childhood but pressure sores may develop in adolescence; if these become sufficiently severe so as to cause extensive loss of skin in the sole of the foot, amputation may be the only solution. It is therefore vital to attempt to obtain a plantigrade foot at an early age.

Some babies are born with established foot deformity. Many birth deformities (*e.g.* pes cavus with claw toes, or calcaneus deformities) are related to intra-uterine paralysis, but it is possible that a few deformities such as talipes equino-varus or convex pes valgus (vertical talus) are associated congenital deformities.

Only a limited amount of correction can be achieved safely by conservative measures such as serial manipulations and plasters, and, even if correction can be achieved, it will not be maintained if there is unbalanced muscle action at the ankle and foot. Operative treatment can be undertaken at any time between the sixth month and second year of life in an attempt to correct deformity and to restore muscle balance. Difficulties in the management of the foot exist not so much in operative technique as in assessment of muscle activity before operation and in deciding upon the best means of producing the balance of muscle action. Even after careful assessment, good correction at the time of operation, and a plantigrade foot immediately after removal of plaster, recurrence of deformity or the development of a new deformity may require a second or even a third corrective procedure.

Assessment should therefore include a detailed analysis of all elements of deformity at the ankle and foot, a testing of clinical muscle activity, and, most important, electrical testing to reveal the existence of all muscles with lower motor neurone innervation. In children below the age of two years, release or elongation of tight muscles and tendons that are producing or maintaining deformity will often give excellent correction without the need to resort to bony procedures and there is often more difficulty with skin closure than with joint mobility.

Plaster fixation after operation is safe provided that the cast is not moulded to attempt to produce more correction than has resulted from the operative division. It is not feasible to describe all the possible variants of tendon transplantation, capsule and ligamentous release, neurectomy, osteotomy or bone excision that can be used to

107

correct a foot deformity. In general, as much correction as possible should first be obtained by division of tendons, ligaments and joint capsules, together with appropriate tendon transplantation or denervations to produce a balance of muscle action at the joints of the ankle and foot. The use of springs to replace weak muscles is also a possible measure (Strach 1972). Procedures involving bone should normally be reserved for a second stage of correction of a deformity that has proved impossible to correct by soft tissue surgery alone.

Equinovarus Deformity

Equinovarus is the most common deformity of the foot in spina bifida (Fig. 10.7). Although a number of variants of pattern of innervation may be present, the common distribution of muscle activity is, as might be expected, associated with prominent action of the invertors and plantar flexors and weakness of the dorsiflexors and evertors.

Elongation of the tendo calcaneus, the tibialis posterior tendon and the long flexor tendons of the toes together with posterior and medial capsulectomy and division of the medial ligaments of the ankle and subtaloid joint gives correction in most instances at any age up to two years. Muscle balance can be restored by lateral transplantation of the tibialis anterior or transplantation of the tibialis posterior tendon through the interosseous membrane to the dorsum and outer side of the foot. The decision as to which transplant is likely to be more appropriate will depend on the analysis of strength of activity in the dorsiflexors and plantar flexors of the ankle and foot.

In some children, equinovarus of the hind-foot is associated with adduction of the fore-foot to such a degree that the line of the fore-foot is 90 degrees medially rotated relative to the plane of the knee joint. An extensive release of the structures on

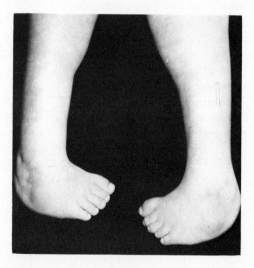

Fig. 10.7. Severe equinovarus deformity due to paralysis of dorsiflexors and evertors.

108

the medial and plantar aspects of the foot will correct much of the metatarsus varus, but if the deformity cannot be corrected completely (especially in a child over the age of 18 months), partial or complete excision of the cuboid (Evans 1961) or a multiple basal osteotomy of the metatarsals (Heyman *et al.* 1958) may be needed to complete correction of deformity. At the hind-foot, if varus deformity has not been able to be corrected completely by soft tissue division, calcaneal osteotomy (Dwyer 1959) to correct varus of the heel may be needed at a second stage. In severe and intractable cases, talectomy may be the only solution (Menelaus 1971*b*).

Occasionally, equinus of the ankle combined with adduction and varus of the fore-foot may be due to reflex activity in the triceps surae and intrinsic foot muscles in the absence of any other active muscles in the limb below the knee. In this situation, a different procedure is required. The tendo calcaneus needs to be elongated and, at the same time, the sole of the foot explored; any tight plantar structures should be released and the nerve supply of the intrinsic muscles divided, either by selective plantar denervation or by division of the main trunk of the posterior tibial nerve. At a second operation six weeks later, half of the tendo calcaneus is transplanted either through the interosseous membrane to the dorsum of the foot or around the outer side of the fibula to the dorsum of the foot. In this way, a muscular tenodesis is produced and recurrent equinus deformity may be prevented.

Calcaneus and Calcaneo-Valgus Deformity

Calcaneus deformities (Fig. 9.3) are less common than equinus deformities but are much commoner than in other varieties of paralytic deformity. Although the patient may be capable of walking in the presence of some calcaneus, the situation is a dangerous one in that excessive pressure on the heel is ultimately likely to give rise to an intractable pressure sore.

The basic requirement is that some power should be diminished from the dorsiflexors and, if necessary, added to that of the plantar flexors. If there is no activity to be found in the triceps surae or any of the other ankle plantar flexors (as shown by a negative response to faradic stimulation) but there is good activity in all the dorsiflexors, transplantation of tibialis anterior and peroneus tertius to the tendo calcaneus through the interosseous membrane, together with lengthening of the remaining tendons as required, will correct deformity and give muscle balance, though very little voluntary activity can be expected and a supporting caliper or brace is likely to be needed.

If there is calcaneovalgus deformity, especially one in which the peroneus brevis is displaced over the lower end of the fibula to become a perverted dorsiflexor, correction needs to be made by elongation of the dorsiflexors and transplantation of the peroneus brevis to the insertion of the tibialis posterior. It may also be necessary to transplant one or more of the dorsiflexor tendons to the tendo calcaneus. Deformity persisting into later childhood may require correction by a special form of two-stage triple arthrodesis of Elmslie (Cholmeley 1953). In this operation, any cavus deformity at the mid-tarsal joint is corrected by a wedge re-section and mid-tarsal arthrodesis, followed six weeks later by arthrodesis of the subtaloid joint through a posterior approach with removal of the wedge base posteriorly.

Paralytic Convex Pes Valgus (Vertical Talus)

This deformity is one in which there is equinovalgus at the hind-foot, calcaneovalgus at the fore-foot, and dislocation at the talonavicular joint (Fig. 9.4). The dorsiflexor tendons are extremely tight and bowstring across the anterior aspect of the ankle, the tibialis posterior is stretched and ineffective, and the intrinsic muscles are paralysed (Drennan and Sharrard 1971, Duckworth and Smith 1974).

Correction needs to be made through two incisions. Through a dorso-medial incision the tibialis anterior is divided from the navicular and medial cuneiform bones, and the toe extensor tendons and peroneus tertius tendons are elongated. This allows the fore-foot to be plantar flexed and the dislocation of the navicular to be reduced onto the head of the talus where it is maintained by a transfixing pin. Through a postero-lateral incision, valgus deformity of the hind-foot is corrected by detachment of the peroneus brevis from its insertion, release of the lateral side of the subtaloid joint, elongation of the tendo calcaneus, and transplantation of the peroneus brevis tendon behind the ankle to the medial side to be attached to the navicular at the insertion of the tibialis posterior. The tibialis anterior tendon is sutured to the neck of the talus. If this operation is done at some time between the sixth and eighteenth month of life, a satisfactory correction can be obtained. An alternative method is one in which all the tight tendons are divided and excised with correction of the deformity and production of a flail foot (Walker and Cheong-Leem 1973).

If correction has not been made before the child is two years old, it is still possible to make a correction in a similar way to those described above except that the navicular may need to be removed.

Pes Cavus and Claw Toes

The mildest form of foot deformity is present when there is paresis of the intrinsic foot muscles but no paralysis in any of the other muscles of the foot. Deformity is not marked (or develops very slowly) and it may at first seem unnecessary to consider any operative correction (Fig. 9.5).

However, the situation is fraught with hazard, since the child is usually very active and there is at least partial loss of sensibility in the toes, or complete loss of sensibility in the fore-foot and toes. Ideally, the deformity is corrected while it is still mobile by release of any tight structures in the sole from the calcaneus to correct any cavus deformity, transplantation of the long flexor tendon in each lesser toe to the dorsum of the toe (Taylor 1951) and a tenodesis of the flexor hallucis longus to the proximal phalanx (Smith and Sharrard 1973), possibly combined with elongation of the extensors of the great toe.

If the child is more than 11 years old, it may not be possible to correct fixed deformity except by bony procedures. These include arthrodesis of one or both interphalangeal joints in each lesser toe and arthrodesis of the interphalangeal joint of the great toe combined with transplantation of the extensor hallucis longus tendon to the neck of the first metatarsal.

Flail Foot

A truly flail foot does not usually develop fixed deformity, but when bearing weight valgus not capable of control by bracing may be present and cause ulceration of the medial malleolus. Supra-malleolar osteotomy of the tibia (see Fig. 10.8 and Sharrard and Webb 1974) or sub-taloid arthrodesis (Grice 1952) or both procedures may be needed. Arthrodesis of the ankle or pan-taloid arthrodesis is contra-indicated (Hayes *et al.* 1964).

MANAGEMENT OF THE SPINE

Kyphosis

Some degree of kyphosis of the lumbar spine is present at birth in one in 20 myelomeningoceles. In some babies, the kyphotic deformity is already severe at birth and with it there is usually severe lower limb paralysis associated with a thin myeloschisis stretched over the apex of the kyphos. In other instances, an acute kyphos at the lumbo-sacral junction may be combined with absence of the sacrum and coccyx. Severe deformity at birth may make surgical closure of the spinal lesion difficult or impossible unless the kyphotic deformity is partially corrected by osteotomy-excision of the spine. This can be performed in the neonate at the same time as closure of the spinal defect (Sharrard 1968). The operation is a severe one, requiring expert anaesthesia and accurate blood replacement. The prognosis for limb function is poor and hydrocephalus is almost invariably present. Thus, although correction of the deformity and primary closure of myelomeningocele defect can be obtained initially, the functional end result several years later is very poor and this category of child may well be one in whom surgical treatment is withheld at birth.

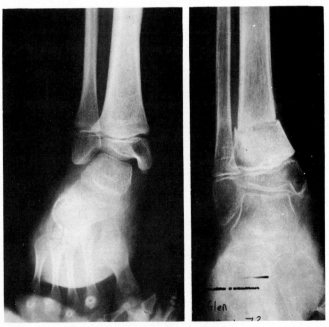

Fig. 10.8. Radiograph of valgus deformity of the ankle in a flail foot: (*left*) before operation; (*right*) after supramalleolar osteotomy of the tibia.

Although milder degrees of kyphos with less severe paralysis may not require correction of the spinal deformity at birth, the deformity does increase in early childhood. Partial lower limb paralysis may increase, the skin over the kyphos may become thin and liable to ulceration, and the fitting of braces becomes progressively more difficult (Fig. 10.9). Unless some surgical action is taken, the end result may be a child with complete lower limb paralysis who is unable to use any kind of brace for walking and is likely to have large ulcers over the projecting spine even when sitting in a special chair. The spine proximal and distal to the kyphos develops a secondary fixed lordosis.

Increasing paralysis, the development of ulceration, or inability to apply bracing, are all indications of the need for correction by excision-osteotomy of the spine (Eyring *et al.* 1972, Sharrard and Drennan 1972).

The apical vertebra (with possibly one or even two vertebrae proximal to it) are removed to allow correction of the prominence of the kyphos (Fig. 10.10). The spine is held with staples or screws and the patient nursed in a plaster bed for three months until union is secure. Removal of the vertebrae does not lead to any decrease in the height of the trunk, since the vertebrae that are removed are those that are projecting posteriorly into the kyphos. Although the operation is a major one, mortality in the older child is minimal and the functional results are satisfactory.

Lordosis and Lordoscoliosis

Lordosis is not seen in spina bifida at birth or in early childhood. In spite of a major defect in the lumbar laminae and spinous processes, many children remain free from significant spinal deformity for the first eight or nine years of life. At about the age of 10 or 11, possibly in relation to the pre-adolescent growth spurt, increasing lordosis associated with scoliosis may develop, particularly in those who have an extensive spinal defect; the situation is worse when there is severe lower limb paralysis with activity only in the hip flexor muscles. Flexion deformity at the hip and the need to sit for long periods in a wheel-chair increase the lordotic tendency (Fig. 10.11). The deformity may make it impossible to wear bracing for walking and may even make sitting in a wheel-chair impossible. Corrective measures by means of plaster casts, polythene supports or Milwaukee braces are difficult to apply and are liable to cause pressure sores in the sacral and iliac regions. As the child becomes older, the heavy weight of the upper trunk causes him to fall forwards into increasing lordosis and no kind of apparatus can sustain the upright position of the trunk: operative treatment alone can provide correction.

A significant amount of correction of deformity can first be achieved by skull-femoral traction using skull calipers or a halo caliper and traction pins through the lower femur with the patient on a Stryker frame. After four to six weeks, surgical correction and fusion of any remaining deformity can be made. The posterior route is difficult and unrewarding because of the presence of scarring posteriorly, the absence of posterior elements for bone fusion and the impossibility of application of fixation such as Harrington rods (Sriram *et al.* 1972). An anterior approach, particularly in the lower thoracic and lumbar spine where the deformity commonly occurs, is the ideal one for this situation. A combined thoraco-lumbar approach by the transpleural, per-diaphragmatic retro-peritoneal approach recommended by Dwyer is very appropriate for this purpose (Fig. 10.12); it allows excision of the intervertebral discs and vertebral end-plates to correct deformity and fixation of the corrected spine by staples and tension cables (Dwyer *et al.* 1969, Baker and Sharrard 1973). After operation, simple nursing on a Stryker frame for 12 weeks gives sound fusion in a very high proportion of patients. By this method, fusion of the spine can be done without undue difficulty from the eighth thoracic to the fourth or even fifth lumbar vertebra. If scoliosis deformity extends proximal to this level, it is usually in an area not associated with spina bifida and can be corrected and fused by a posterior approach and fusion as in other types of scoliosis.

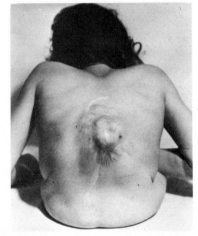

Fig. 10.9 (*right*). Severe progressive lumbar kyphosis.
Fig. 10.10 (*below*). Radiographs of lumbar kyphosis: (*left*) before operation; (*right*) after osteotomy-excision of lumbar vertebrae.

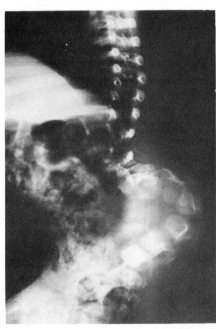
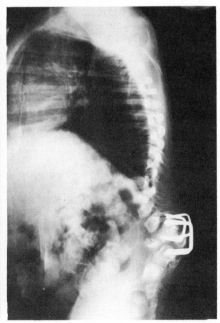

113

Hemivertebrae and Congenital Scoliosis

Spina bifida is frequently accompanied by abnormal vertebral formation. Hemivertebrae (sometimes multiple) in association with fused segments on the opposite side of the spine, and with absent or fused ribs and thoracic and abdominal defects may occur (Fig. 10.13). Hemimyelocele, in which one lower limb is normally innervated and the other is partially paralysed (Fig. 10.14) with asymmetrical myelomeningocele, is almost always associated with hemivertebrae formation and scoliosis (Duckworth *et al.* 1968).

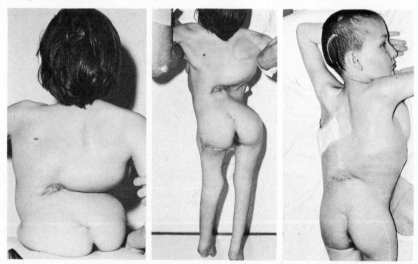

Fig. 10.11. Collapsing type of lordoscoliosis: (*left*) the rib cage overlaps the iliac crest, and pelvic obliquity cuases the patient to sit with her weight on the left ischial tuberosity; (*middle*) slight correction on suspension; (*right*) clinical correction four days after operation. (From Baker and Sharrard 1973.)

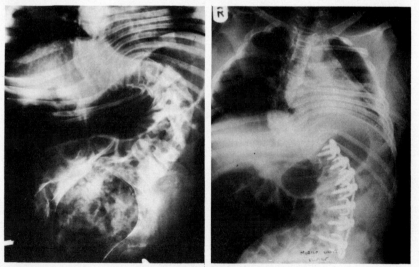

Fig. 10.12. Radiographs of lordoscoliosis (*left*) before, and (*right*) after correction and fusion. Same child as in Fig. 11. (From Baker and Sharrard 1973.)

114

If there are several hemivertebrae, scoliosis may be present at birth. In other instances, scoliosis is not particularly noticeable in infancy but becomes gradually more apparent during childhood. The liability to progressive deformity varies considerably and is not necessarily related to the number of hemivertebrae present. The effects of progressive scoliosis differ in different regions of the spine. Congenital hemivertebra formation in the uppermost part of the thoracic spine gives rise to a very ugly deformity with an elevation of the shoulder. Deformity in the thoracic spine produces a scoliosis comparable to that of idiopathic scoliosis of other types and scoliosis in the lumbar spine is likely to be associated with lordosis and with tilting of the pelvis.

If the state of the skin innervation allows it, it may be possible to use Milwaukee bracing to minimise the progressive development of deformity; if this is not feasible, a rapidly progressing deformity that has increased beyond 45 degrees may need operative treatment at an early age. Fusion of vertebral bodies on the convex edge of the curve can be made at any age between three and 10 years and may succeed in preventing the progress of further deformity. Anterior or posterior correction and fusion can then be made.

Excision osteotomy of a hemivertebra is a major procedure requiring removal of vertebral body anteriorly and any posterior processes posteriorly. Considerable care needs to be exercised to avoid damage to the spinal cord or to the arteries supplying it, but in severe deformity its performance may be justifiable.

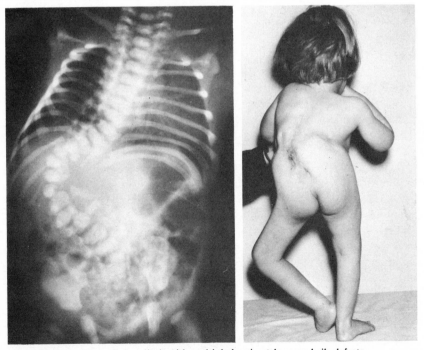

Fig. 10.13 (*left*). Congenital scoliosis with multiple hemivertebrae and rib defects.
Fig. 10.14 (*right*). Hemimyelocele. The right lower limb is normal and the left lower limb is paralysed. There is scoliosis with hemivertebrae.

THE MANAGEMENT OF COMPLICATIONS OF SENSORY LOSS

Pressure Sores

Pressure sores usually occur in an area of anaesthetic skin that is subject to pressure or friction and overlying a bony prominence. Thus, the important areas that may develop pressure sores include the plantar surface of the foot, the ischial tuberosities, the outer side of the hips, or the front of the knees.

A completely anaesthetic sole will sustain the pressures of weight-bearing provided that the pressure is distributed evenly and the degree of pressure (as represented by the area of the sole of the foot in relation to the weight of the child) is acceptable.

A much more important measure in the prevention of pressure sores in the sole of the foot is the prevention of fixed deformity. Minor degrees of varus, valgus, calcaneus or equinus are acceptable for bearing weight in poliomyelitis or cerebral palsy but are not tolerated by the anaesthetic foot. An additional problem is that whilst the foot may tolerate some deformity during childhood, the increase in weight of the child in adolescence without concomitant growth of the size of the foot is very likely to result in development of pressure sores for the first time after the age of 10 years. Ideally, all deformities which might give rise to high points of pressure in the sole of the foot should have been corrected by the time the child is five or six years of age. If, by the age of 10 or 11 years, there is evidence suggesting some persistent deformity and high spots of pressure, a final correction by bony operation or triple arthrodesis is indicated.

The more active the child, and the better his general level of innervation at the lower limbs, the more likelihood there is for pressure sores in the feet to develop because of the degree of activity that the child can achieve. A child with no innervation below the second sacral segment is often in danger of pressure ulceration in the toes; the toes may become clawed and, failing correction, pressure ulceration develops at the tips with secondary sepsis leading to the need to amputate the toe and sometimes several toes in succession.

The parents must be taught to look for any areas of excessive redness on the soles of the child's feet, as these might betoken the early development of pressure sores. The older child must be taught to inspect the soles of his feet regularly by the use of a mirror. Boots and shoes need to be fitted well and are useful in spreading pressure evenly in the sole of the foot. In cold weather, fleece-lined boots have a dual advantage of preventing chilblains and avoiding excessive pressure.

Ischial sores are likely to arise in children who are severely paralysed and confined to a wheel-chair. Flexion deformity at the hips or lordoscoliosis in the lumbar spine increase the liability to ischial pressure sores. The child needs to be taught to alter the distribution of weight regularly from one buttock to another or from one area of skin to another. The child and parents must be taught that the child should not be allowed to sit on a hard surface for longer than a few minutes at a time. Where possible, the application of calipers to allow a child to stand for several periods during a day to relieve pressure on the buttock skin is an important prophylactic measure.

Pressure ulceration on the front of the knees occurs in younger children as a result of crawling on their knees, or, in the case of severely paralysed lower limbs, dragging themselves along in the prone position. The supply of calipers to produce upright weight-bearing will usually allow these sores to heal. The problem seldom exists in older children.

Pressure sores can also arise within plaster casts, especially when the casts are used in an attempt to correct fixed deformity. However, provided the casts are applied carefully and evenly with a layer of plaster wool that is not too thin or too thick, it should be possible to avoid these pressure sores. A plaster cast that is too loose may be an even more pertinent cause of ulceration due to friction inside the cast, especially in an active child capable of bearing weight on the cast. When a hip spica is required for the correction of deformities in the proximal part of the lower limbs, the cast should always include the paralysed feet. If the cast ends at ankle level, there is considerable liability to pressure ulceration at the back of the ankle over the tendo calcaneus.

Calipers can also be a source of pressure ulceration, especially at the knee. If there is flexion or varus or valgus deformity at the knee and attempts are made to hold the limb in the corrected position by means of straps and pads, a pressure sore can easily result if there is a fixed deformity. Ring-top or ischial-weight-bearing calipers are likely to produce pressure sores in the perineum and ischial region and are best avoided in children with spina bifida.

Skin ulceration in the perineum and ischial region is often aggravated by persistent wetness due to incontinence of urine and/or faeces.

Most pressure sores will heal if the cause of pressure is removed, the area is kept free of pressure for sufficiently long, and simple measures taken to protect the sores from serious infection. The application of topical antibiotics is seldom useful, especially if a child is allowed to bear weight on an ulcerated area. If infection does occur, it is better to treat it with a systemic antibiotic.

Very serious problems may arise in relation to pressure sores in two sites, *i.e.* on the plantar surface of the heel or in relation to the ischial tuberosities. If a heel sore results in complete loss of the whole of the thickness of the healed skin directly on the weight-bearing area of the heel, it is very likely that the limb will have to be amputated. No kind of skin graft or pedicle graft can replace heel skin; the moment the child starts to bear weight on the limb again, the heel will break down very rapidly. Even if an amputation is performed, the flaps of the amputation stump must be so made as to provide skin with sensibility over the end of the stump.

Ischial or sacral pressure sores are likely to become serious problems if extensive necrosis of the fatty and subcutaneous tissues occurs with extensive undermining and even more so if the ischial tuberosity itself becomes infected. An extensive period lying prone to avoid pressure on the area may allow healing to occur but recurrent breakdown is common and sometimes only an extensive skin flap taken from an innervated area of the back will allow permanent healing.

Abnormal responses to cold make chilblains a common problem in limbs that are unprotected from cold weather, but these will usually heal once the cold weather ceases.

Gangrene of the skin of the foot and toes may result from excessive exposure to cold. The child should not be allowed to walk about in snow, even when wearing

117

adequate footwear. The feet may be burned or scalded by the injudicious use of hot water bottles or on contact with a hot radiator.

Spontaneous Fractures

Pathological fractures are liable to occur in the bones of the lower limbs in spina bifida patients (James 1970). There is a general relationship between the liability to fracture and the extent of paralysis, so that children with complete flaccid lower limb paralysis are much more likely to develop fractures than those with minimal paralysis or reflex innervation. There is also some relationship between the level of paralysis and the level at which fractures may occur. In limbs with complete paralysis, fractures may occur at any part of the femur or tibia. In children with innervation down to the third lumbar segment, the commonest site for fracture is the lower end of the femur or upper end of the tibia; when innervation exists down to the fifth lumbar or first sacral segment, fractures are likely to occur at the lower end of the tibia or in the foot. The factors that relate to the liability to spontaneous fractures are probably multiple. Paralysis and disuse make the limb bones slender and porotic (Alliaume 1950). Sensory loss may contribute in some undefined way to the quality of the bone. Lack of sensibility in the periosteum and soft tissues adds to the liability to fracture because of the absence of pain when the bone is put under excessive stress, *e.g.* when a child gets his legs between the bars of a cot and wriggles or turns over. Immobilisation in plaster following an operation (*e.g.* operations on the hip) is especially liable to lead to increased osteoporosis and bone fragility; special care needs to be taken to try to prevent minor trauma to the limb that might lead to a fracture during the first three or four weeks following removal of a plaster cast.

There may be additional metabolic causes for bone fragility such as renal rickets due to disturbance of vitamin D metabolism by renal failure or renal abnormality, and this is particularly liable to give rise to a displaced upper femoral or lower femoral epiphysis. Abnormal utilisation of vitamin C has also been implicated as a cause of spontaneous epiphyseal separations (McKibbin and Porter 1967, McKibbin *et al.* 1968).

The diagnosis of spontaneous fracture in spina bifida is often missed by those unaware of the characteristic signs. There is seldom any history of injury. The affected portion of the limb becomes swollen and slightly warm but is completely painless. There is often a mild general pyrexia which may reach as high as 39 degrees and blood investigations may show a raised erythrocyte sedimentation rate and white cell count. If the fracture occurs near the bone end, it may not be possible to detect abnormal mobility; radiological changes may be almost undetectable at first, especially in a slight fracture-separation of the lower femoral or upper or lower tibial epiphysis. For all these reasons, the lesion is very commonly treated as an osteomyelitis with the administration of antibiotics which are, naturally, ineffective. After four or five days, a further radiological examination reveals extensive new bone formation characteristic of a fracture in spina bifida due to extensive sub-periosteal haemorrhage and laying down of bone (Fig. 10.15). Unfortunately, during this period the epiphysis may displace, resulting in genu valgum or genu varum, or valgus or varus deformities of the ankle. At the hip, the upper femoral epiphysis may slip and result in a coxa vara with or without avascular necrosis of the upper femoral epiphysis. Fractures of the shaft of the bone, particularly the femur, occur slightly less commonly, but once a fracture of this kind has occurred the bone that results following union of the fracture is often persistently abnormal and there is yet further liability to another fracture. Occasionally, a recurrent sequence of fractures may occur so that as many as twelve fractures may occur in succession in the same bone. This is particularly likely to occur when the general health of the child is poor and a severe state of osteoporosis has developed.

The treatment of pathological fractures in spina bifida should be the minimum possible necessary to maintain alignment of the limb. Union of the fractured bone occurs so rapidly in younger children that the fracture has often united by the time it has been diagnosed.

For fractures of the shaft of the femur, traction in a Thomas splint should be avoided; the counter pressure of the ring of the splint in the groin inevitably produces serious pressure sores. There is seldom any need for traction, especially if the limb is paralysed, and simple multiple wool and crêpe bandages are often all that is required to maintain alignment. If traction is required, it should be free traction with the limb on a pillow. For fractures at the knee, a groin-to-ankle plaster cast can be used for a few days, and for fractures at the lower end of the tibia a below-knee plaster cast may be required, but only for a short time.

Charcot Joints

The joints of children with spina bifida are not subject to progressive degenerative change in infancy or early childhood but degeneration may be seen in older children, especially those in whom paralysis is relatively slight or present only in one limb. The commonest place for the development of a Charcot joint in childhood is at the subtaloid joint, secondary to pathological fractures of the calcaneum and the talus. Disintegration of the talus may in turn lead to a type of Charcot joint at the ankle. Large fragments of articular cartilage at the knee and portions of the bone of the femoral condyle may become detached, causing locking and early osteoarthritis in the knee joint. For these reasons, children with minimal paralysis but with sensory loss in one or more joints in one limb should not undertake active sports, particularly contact sports.

PROBLEMS OF LOCOMOTION

Each individual spina bifida child is likely to have a somewhat different set of problems in attempting to gain independence in walking. There are four main factors in locomotion in spina bifida:—
(1) The level and nature of innervation of the lower limbs.
(2) The presence of hydrocephalus.
(3) The presence of deformity and the feasibility of bracing.
(4) Intelligence.

The level of motor innervation of the lower limbs determines the extent of bracing that is likely to be needed. In general, if there is good innervation from all lumbar segments, braces will only be needed below knee level. If there is innervation from the first four lumbar segments, bracing will only be needed below knee level provided that stabilising procedures such as postero-lateral iliopsoas transplants have been done at the hip level. Paralysis greater than this almost always requires bracing at hip, knee and foot, as does any limb with reflex paralysis or autonomous muscle activity only. If intelligence is normal and there is no hydrocephalus, any spina bifida child should be able to become independent in walking provided that appropriate bracing has been applied and deformity has been corrected, since the trunk musculature is almost always sufficient to elevate the pelvis to allow alternate limbs to clear the ground.

Significant hydrocephalus and diminished intelligence (which often occur together) render independent walking much more difficult, whatever the degree of lower limb paralysis. Hydrocephalus disturbs balance and spatial orientation so that, even if there is very little paralysis in the lower limbs, a child with hydrocephalus has difficulty in balancing until he is more than four or five years old and is very frightened of attempting to walk across a space unless he is touching another individual by the hand or has some means of guidance by the upper limbs. If intelligence is poor, the child will not be able to work out how to use his limbs and how to make use of any apparatus to propel himself.

In preparation for walking, an infant can be placed in various positions to improve his balance and encourage him to roll over, to reach for playthings and to play with toys of increasing weight. Training methods are employed to improve strength in shoulder girdle and arm muscles, including activities such as wheelbarrow races, push-ups, and propulsion using a low four-wheel trolley.

When the child is about a year old, at about the time when he might usually start to walk, the use of a standing frame or one of its variants such as a parapodium can be used to enable the child to become accustomed to being in the vertical position (Paul 1972). Many small children are able to make excellent use of a swivel walking apparatus which relies on rotary movements of the trunk for forward propulsion. This device becomes less useful when the child becomes older and heavier, although it has the advantage that the child is able to use its arms freely and does not require any help from crutches or sticks.

Double calipers and trunk support with hip hinges (Fig. 10.16) allowing 20 degrees of abduction and adduction and a small free range of flexion and extension (Fig. 10.17) make it possible for even a severely paralysed child to walk with an alternate gait using a walking frame and later elbow crutches (Herzog and Sharrard 1966). Less severely paralysed children may be able to discard the hip support when walking balance is well established and to progress with gradually less apparatus depending on the degree of paralysis that exists.

Many children can progress much more rapidly with the help of a swing-through gait and crutches. Although the appearance is not so elegant, the child can progress with considerable speed and can even play games such as football using this mechanism. It should not therefore be discouraged but the child should be taught alternate lower limb walking as well.

As the child comes towards puberty, it becomes more and more difficult to sustain walking ability, especially in children who are severely paralysed. The size of the apparatus required, the increase in weight without commensurate increase in muscle power in the lower limbs at the time of the pubertal growth spurt and a tendency to obesity all tend to make a child more and more dependent on a wheel-chair. Although this may be to some extent inevitable, there are a number of important disadvantages to a wheel-chair existence:—

(1) There is a considerable tendency to obesity and the development of oedema of the lower limbs with laying down of fibro-fatty tissue.

(2) Porosis of the lower limb bones makes fractures more likely to occur.

(3) Unless great care is taken, ischial sores may develop and if a deep and intractable ischial sore develops, it may be impossible to resume even wheel-chair locomotion.

(4) The ureters may be kinked and aggravate a liability to hydronephrosis, especially if there is lordosis of the lumbar spine.

Even if a child does have to use a wheel-chair for the majority of the time, an attempt to walk should be made each day so as to maintain such lower limb function as is present, to try to maintain strength in the lower limb bones, to relieve pressure on the ischial region, to allow the bladder to drain properly and to use up surplus calories to minimise obesity.

Special types of calipers have been devised to aid independent walking, particularly in those children who have good flexor power but absent extension at the hip. The use of a link between the two limbs with a gear box such that flexion of one limb produces extension of the opposite limb has a useful place in children with paralysis below the second or third lumbar segment.

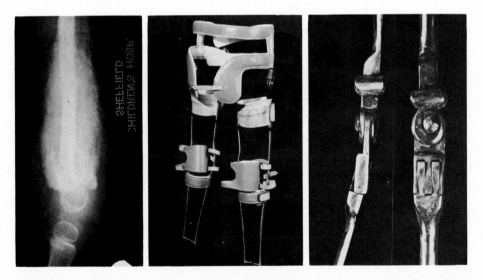

Fig. 10.15 (*left*). Hyperplastic callus formation in association with spontaneous fracture of the lower end of the femur.

Fig. 10.16 (*middle*). Double calipers with trunk support for extensive paralysis.

Fig. 10.17 (*right*). Semi-mobile hip hinges for use in association with double calipers and trunk support, allowing a limited range of free abduction and adduction for alternate gait walking.

CHAPTER 11

Management of Bladder and Bowel in Spina Bifida

D. Forrest

Introduction

Since the urinary tract and bowel are involved in 90 per cent of spina bifida aperta cases (see Chapter 4) and in a significant number of cases where the spinal defect is less obvious (see Chapter 7), its management is an important part of the total care of spina bifida. Although Tribe (1963) found the cause of death to be pyelonephritis in 44 per cent of cases of acquired paraplegia coming to autopsy, this does not seem to apply to spina bifida: Laurence (1964) found the cause of death to be renal failure in only four per cent of untreated cases, whilst Eckstein *et al.* (1967) found only three per cent in untreated cases and nine per cent in treated cases.

In terms of quality of survival, proper urological management clearly has much to offer by avoidance of chronic ill-health and social ostracism. If this aspect of the disorder is taken care of from birth, most, but not all, deaths from renal causes should be avoidable.

Although much can be learnt from the vast literature on acquired paraplegia in adults, it is important to remember that only a minority of spina bifida patients have such a straightforward neurological picture (Chapter 4). Experience with spina bifida treated intensively from birth in the past 15 years is now producing a considerable volume of experience in its own right.

Normal and Abnormal Micturition

Normal micturition and the acquisition of continence are due to an extremely subtle combination of neurophysiology, hydrodynamics and psychology, and are still very imperfectly understood.

Intermittent filling and emptying of the bladder begins as early as the third month of fetal life and continues after birth until maturational development of the supra-segmental pathways, both facilitatory and inhibitory, permits increasing control by day and night, but, even then, the pattern of complete dryness, then a steady, powerful stream until the bladder is empty, followed once more by dryness without dribbling, continues. In a normal infant the bladder cannot be emptied by external pressure except when under general anaesthetic.

Normal continence is not dependent on the external urethral sphincter which is a second line of defence. Debate about the rôle of the internal sphincter continues, but it is clear that the bladder neck, when at rest, is closed (Hutch 1971). Tone in the muscles of the pelvic floor keeps the bladder neck elevated. Vincent (1966) has shown that until the bladder neck descends, micturition is impossible.

By the age of four or five years the normal individual has acquired all the characteristics of adult micturition, namely:

(1) Intermittent awareness of the bladder as it contracts, at first tentatively and quickly suppressed, but later more insistent.

(2) Ability to realise the state of fullness and plan ahead to a convenient time to go to the lavatory.

(3) Ability to inhibit early contractions and postpone micturition, but to facilitate the emptying reflex when circumstances are right, even when the bladder is only partly full.

(4) Awareness that the bladder has emptied completely.

(5) Ability to withstand emptying when overfilled, or during momentary stress, by voluntary tightening of the pelvic floor and external sphincter.

(6) Ability to stop—though with some difficulty—the flow of urine in mid-stream.

(7) Ability to inhibit emptying during sleep.

The normal adult can initiate micturition when the bladder contains only 30ml, yet at other times the bladder can contain over a litre and can be emptied until it contains less than five ml of residual urine.

Abnormal micturition varies with the nature of the denervation and is modified by overdistension and infection. The completely denervated bladder retains its natural intrinsic contractility, but this is unco-ordinated and insufficient to empty the bladder adequately. The pattern which emerges in spina bifida depends on the state of the bladder neck and posterior urethra, which may stay wide open, and the external sphincter and pelvic floor, which may tighten involuntarily or be partly or completely flaccid.

A mildly affected patient may suffer only some diurnal urgency and nocturnal enuresis, while a more severely paralysed patient may be continent except for occasional stress incontinence.

The majority of spina bifida patients have a fairly capacious bladder which empties partially in spurts or dribbles, mainly as a result of external pressures such as abdominal contraction and changes in posture or manual expression. In these patients there is a serious risk of infection and renal damage, for there is usually no sensation of fullness or emptying, and only occasionally is abdominal pain with over-distension experienced. A few patients have an almost empty dribbling bladder, and in these there is usually no urine to express unless the patient has been lying supine for a while.

A spina bifida infant with an efficient reflex bladder may appear to perform normally until the age is reached when voluntary control should be attained. It then becomes increasingly obvious that the patient lacks the normal sensation of a full bladder and cannot consciously stop or start the flow. Since his reflex emptying depends on complex co-ordination of detrusor, sphincters and pelvic floor it is rarely satisfactory, and consists of partial, unheralded emptying with no long periods of dryness. Manual expression is not possible in these patients unless they can be persuaded to lie down and relax.

In most cases the abnormal pattern of micturition remains unaltered. There is a general tendency for a sphincter which has at first appeared flaccid to become increasingly spastic so that expression becomes increasingly difficult. Occasionally a patient experiences a gradual or sudden change in sensation or control. The change may be for the worse, such as that due to progressive denervation or chronic cystitis, or, surprisingly, after five years or more, sensation may be appreciated or voluntary emptying become possible for the first time.

Clinical Types

Clinicians have always found difficulty in classifying types of neurogenic bladder. This is understandable when one considers the huge number of possible combinations of neurological deficit in the bladder, sphincters and pelvic floor—motor and sensory, somatic and splanchnic, upper or lower motor neurone, complete or patchy, and with changes occurring as the result of infection or obstruction. Although it is not difficult to define broad categories, it is always surprising how different centres find very different types of lesion predominating. For instance, Roberts (1962) described five types, three of them with an active detrusor, and Stark (1973) calculated that two thirds of cases would have an active bladder, while Smith (1965) found an active detrusor 'excessively unusual', and in most of his cases found a low-capacity, easily expressible bladder.

The state of the lower urinary tract is determined by the detrusor tone, which also decides the state of the bladder neck and activity of the external urethral sphincter and levator ani. The interaction of these over a period of time, including fetal life, makes the bladder small and contracted, flaccid and smooth, or, large, thick-walled and trabeculated.

No classification will cover every possible combination, but a simple grouping related to the clinical types described in Chapter 4 is suggested.

GROUP I: Complete or mixed upper motor neurone lesion, corresponding to Types 1 and 3 in Chapter 4.

The bladder is of normal size, sometimes smooth but usually trabeculated. Expulsive detrusor contractions are strong but not well co-ordinated. The sphincters can contract tightly but are not under normal voluntary control. Manual expression produces a stream when the patient is relaxed but stops abruptly when the abdominal muscles tighten up or the child cries. The upper tract may be normal but tends to become dilated in time.

GROUP II: Incomplete lower motor neurone lesion, corresponding to Type 4 in Chapter 4.

The bladder is of normal or above-normal capacity, smooth-walled or trabeculated. Detrusor contractions are weak and intravesical pressure is low. There is sufficient outflow resistance to keep the patient dry until the bladder contains a considerable volume of urine. There is tone in the external urethral and anal sphincters, but this is less than normal. The bladder is expressible. The upper tract dilates early with reflux and recurrent infection.

GROUP III: Complete lower motor neurone lesion, corresponding to Type 2 in Chapter 4.

The bladder is smooth and of normal or small size. The sphincters are conspicuously patulous. Urine dribbles constantly except when the patient is supine and the bladder is empty. The upper tract remains normal and infection is not a problem. This group is the least common.

Relation to Neurological Lesion

Kirkland (1962), Eckstein (1968) and Lister (1969) found it impossible to correlate bladder function with neurological level or lower limb activity. It is certainly more difficult in spina bifida than in acquired paraplegia, partly because of the complexity of the cord lesion and also because of secondary factors modifying behaviour from before birth. However, Stark (1968, 1973) has been able to show a clear correlation between detrusor activity and the neurological level in the lower limbs, though not a very close link with the vertebral level: such a correlation should be of great value when assessing an infant at birth for giving a prognosis for continence and renal function (see Chapters 4 and 6).

Associated Malformations of the Urinary Tract

Malformations of the urinary tract are among the commonest in the otherwise normal population. Wilcox and Emery (1970) found 5.3 per cent in patients dying of other causes but 29 per cent in myelomeningocele deaths. Smith (1965) found nine associated dysplasias in 64 spina bifida patients (14 per cent), besides 34 abnormalities such as mega-ureter, hydronephrosis and vesico-ureteric reflux, most of which could be considered as results of bladder dysfunction, though some were found to have anatomical malformation of the uretero-vesical junction. Forbes *et al.* (1969) studied the intrinsic innervation of dilated ureters in spina bifida, but found no deficiency in either adrenergic or cholinergic supply.

Some associated anomalies such as solitary kidney may result from abnormal bladder function in early fetal life, while others, especially crossed ectopia, are seen mainly in cases with kyphotic thoraco-lumbar spines or hemi-vertebra, and have presumably arisen as a by-product of gross malformation of the vertebral column.

Progressive Pathology

Mechanisms

Inefficient bladder emptying is responsible for almost the whole range of progressive deterioration in the urinary tract. An active detrusor, contracting inefficiently or against an unsynchronised sphincter ('sphincter-detrusor dyssynergia'), hypertrophies and the bladder becomes sacculated or diverticular. Juxta-ureteric diverticula may distort the ureteric tunnel, permitting vesico-ureteric reflux. The bladder neck and external sphincter also thicken, increasing outflow resistance. If such a bladder becomes severely obstructed, dilatation and atony will result.

Incomplete emptying with residual urine of more than about 30ml makes recurrent infection inevitable. Epithelial oedema and hypertrophy, especially in the trigonal area, increase outflow obstruction and interfere with the efficiency of the uretero-vesical valvular mechanism.

An incompletely denervated bladder with poor contractions but nevertheless a relative outflow obstruction also has residual urine and is prone to infection. In this type, ureteric reflux results from paralysis of the muscle embracing the ureter as well as infection. Only the completely denervated system which does not encourage stagnation is reasonably safe from progressive deterioration.

Apart from reflux, upper tract dilatation may be due to mechanical obstruction or prolonged, high intra-vesical pressure in excess of the normal pelvi-ureteric pressure preventing urine from entering the bladder.

Attacks of pyelo-nephritis often occur before there is any radiological evidence of upper tract dilatation, but it is probable that drainage from the pelvis has already been impaired by back-pressure or reflux. By the time reflux can be demonstrated there is already parenchymal damage to the kidneys, and, unless efficient drainage is promptly established, loss of cortex will proceed to eventual renal failure.

Quite apart from anatomical or functional abnormalities of the renal tract, the spina bifida patient is more susceptible to urinary infection than a normal person. Fluid intake may be diminished by the vomiting of raised intra-cranial pressure, sweating due to fever, or voluntary fluid restriction in a misguided attempt to improve continence. Spina bifida patients need a generous fluid intake at all times to maintain a good urinary flow. Lack of exercise leads to stasis in the bladder and the upper tract if it is dilated, and this tendency is most marked when the patient is immobilised prone or head-down for orthopaedic reasons.

Infection

Lorber *et al.* (1968) found 50 per cent of all spina bifida infants to have infected urine before their first birthday. Only about 25 per cent of all cases never develop infections. These are mostly patients with normal pyelograms, although many of them are incontinent.

Routine urine testing shows that half of all patients show significant growth ($> 10^3$/ml) of organisms, usually coliforms, and usually with few pus cells (< 3/mm^3) and accompanied by no local or general symptoms. Such patients have frank infections from time to time, sometimes coming on for obvious reasons—such as during an episode of dehydration—but often arising spontaneously. The pyelogram may be normal, but there is more often dilatation of the upper tract.

About 25 per cent have a continuous urinary infection with opportunist organisms such as Ps.pyocyanea, Proteus or Candida albicans and with numerous pus cells. The urine can be sterilised by the use of the most powerful antibiotics (Lorber and Formby 1968, Holt and Newman 1972), but quickly relapses after the end of the course, in spite of drainage or diversion procedures, no doubt due to persistence of pockets in the damaged renal parenchyma.

Reflux

Whether reflux results from inflammatory oedema, diverticula or paralysis of the uretero-vesical musculature, the effect is progressive dilatation and elongation of the ureters, often one side before the other. Contractions of the ureter, though they may be vigorous, cease to be propulsive. Urine stagnates and becomes permanently infected. Although early hydro-ureter may be seen with an apparently normal pelvis and calyces, it is not long before back pressure and infection, by interference with the blood supply of the renal parenchyma, cause thinning of the renal cortex and hydronephrosis.

Obstruction

Obstruction of the outflow tract is a relative matter, its effect depending on intravesical pressure as much as the numerous intrinsic factors. A few infants develop acute retention within a few days of birth. This may be due to changing condition of the neural plaque causing reflex tightening of the external sphincter. Neglect at this stage will pave the way for irreversible damage to the upper tract. More usual is a gradual chronic retention, with overflow causing gradual deterioration of the bladder and upper tract. From the age of five years or so, an increasing number of patients with an upper motor neurone lesion lose the ability to empty the bladder by manual expression. The external sphincter goes into uncontrollable spasm and urine will pass only if the patient can be persuaded to relax.

Calculus formation

Although n any of the conditions favourable to stone formation (*e.g.* infection, stasis and biochemical imbalance) exist in the urinary tract in spina bifida, this is in fact an extremely rare complication. In well over 1,000 cases the writer has seen only seven patients with stone. Three of these were large bladder stones, one was in the posterior urethra, one was in an ileal loop, one in a defunctioned bladder and one was a staghorn calculus in a patient on skeletal traction with extreme angulation of the bed. This staghorn calculus dissolved spontaneously when the patient was mobilised, and all the others were dealt with easily, so there does not seem to be any need for special safeguards to prevent stones from forming.

Hypertension

Hypertension is a sign of advancing renal damage. It may be the first evidence and should be looked for, especially after the end of the first decade: it is very rarely found before this time. No doubt caused by the parenchymal damage of chronic pyelonephritis, it is a curiously inconstant accompaniment of renal damage in children, being found in only about 10 per cent of cases (Kimmel 1942). Like renal failure, hypertension often becomes worse during attacks of infection, and abates when the infection is controlled.

Renal rickets

In spite of the biochemical disturbances suffered by many spina bifida patients with advancing renal disease, the reported incidence of renal rickets is not high. It is probably present more often than suspected, however. Its appearance may be masked by the more usual bone changes of the paralysed lower limbs, *e.g.* osteoporosis, pathological fractures and joint destruction, and so the wrists and hands (almost the only parts of the skeleton not routinely studied in spina bifida) should be examined for the pathognomonic x-ray changes (Fig. 11.1).

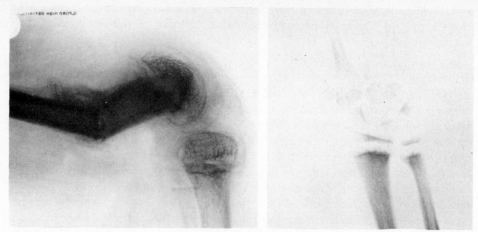

Fig. 11.1 (*left*). Gross bone changes round the knee attributed to paralytic osteoporosis (*Right*) Wrist of same patient showing severe renal tickets.

Renal failure

A severe acute attack of pyelonephritis may cause depression of renal function. In a young child this may be rapid and profound, but equally rapid recovery may take place. In older patients deterioration is likely to be slower but more permanent. Few patients die of renal failure in their first decade, but, after this age, a high proportion do. Free drainage of urine may halt this deterioration in its early stages, but once dilatation and tortuosity of the upper tract become severe, not even supra-vesical diversion will permit a return to normal. It may occasionally be justified to reverse temporary renal failure in an otherwise favourable case by means of peritoneal dialysis, but long-term dialysis or renal transplant are quite out of the question because of the presence of infection, as well as the ethical considerations.

Whereas the normal upper tract permits very little reabsorption of urinary constituants back into the blood stream, the grossly tortuous ureter offers a much less efficient epithelial barrier; it thus adds to the burden of already damaged kidneys by reabsorption, especially of chloride ions.

Orchitis

Unco-ordinated emptying of the bladder, with injudicious attempts at manual expression in the presence of a distal obstruction, may cause reflux of infected urine into the vas deferens, giving rise to recurrent attacks of acute epididymo-orchitis. Since the testis has a sensory nerve supply from L1-2, patients with a low spinal lesion will suffer pain. Inflammation may go on to suppuration and scrotal fistula formation, or recurrent minor attacks may cause fibrosis and atrophy. Vasectomy may be necessary to stop the attacks.

Neonatal Management

Initial assessment

The general initial examination of the infant (see Chapter 6), the level and nature of the neural plaque, and inspection and stimulation of the anal sphincter combine to give a good indication of the innervation of the bladder and whether the external sphincter will be normal, flaccid or spastic. The most revealing part of the examination is the observation of the pattern of unaided micturition, especially whether a considerable volume of urine is passed with force while the infant is lying quietly or whether it dribbles when the baby cries. To this end, the infant should be watched lying naked in an incubator. The neonatal bladder being an abdominal organ, it is easy to assess its size, shape, and resistance to manual expression. At this age, expression is usually best achieved by squeezing the organ transversely between finger and thumb. In a Group II lesion (see page 124) urine dribbles or spurts when the bladder is squeezed, stops when pressure is released, and recommences on further squeezing. This behaviour must be distinguished from that of a normal or a spastic (Group I) bladder which may be triggered by external pressure but then continues to empty after pressure is released. Although it may be expected to empty fully, a spastic bladder seldom does so efficiently, and a firm rounded mass can be felt in the lower abdomen. Even firm pressure produces only a reluctant trickle or nothing at all. A few cases of this type develop acute retention in the neonatal period.

It is probably safest to assume that an infant with sensory or motor deficit in the lower limbs at birth will not have completely normal bladder function, although this is not to say that it will not achieve control.

Smith (1965) found close correlation between perineal sensation and bladder function. If there is saddle anaesthesia, then there is almost certain to be some disturbance of the bladder. Again, however, such patients sometimes achieve control. The converse rule, that normal perineal sensation denotes normal bladder function, has, unfortunately, many exceptions.

Investigations

Infection may become established within a few days of birth, so regular collection of urine specimens for culture and cell count is most important. After cleansing and drying the penis or vulva, a clean urine specimen can be collected either by expression, or, if this is not possible, by applying a length of Paul's tubing or a disposable plastic 'Uribag'. Since contamination is inevitable, it is essential that the specimen should be plated out or refrigerated within minutes of collection. At this age, suprapubic puncture is the easiest and only certain way of collecting an uncontaminated specimen (Nelson and Peters 1965).

Excretion pyelography, if skilfully performed, nearly always gives an excellent picture of the whole urinary tract, and should be performed in the first few weeks of life. If the back has been closed surgically it is wise to defer the examination until the wound has healed soundly. A scalp vein is nearly always available for puncture, and it should not be necessary to resort to a subcutaneous injection. Bladder films allow a good estimate of capacity and show the presence of sacculation or diverticula. If the bladder is expressible, a post-expression film shows how well the bladder empties and the appearance of the outflow tract (Fig. 11.2). If this film is taken after most of the dye has been cleared by the kidneys, it also gives a good guide as to the presence of reflux. Thus, there is seldom any need for a micturating cysto-urethrogram at this age.

In many neonates there is already evidence of outflow obstruction, with an enlarged sacculated bladder. Ureters are often beginning to dilate, but it is uncommon to see severe hydronephrosis at birth.

Management

The first essential is to identify and treat those cases liable to acute retention and thus avoid permanent upper tract damage. A palpable bladder should be expressed regularly. Though this would be done ideally at approximately the normal time intervals for the age (say half-hourly), this would allow the infant too little rest, so a routine of expression at the beginning and end of each feed is an adequate compromise. A bladder which is not expressible may be normal, spastic or empty. If spastic, it is at risk and should be watched, especially for the first few days after back closure, as this often precipitates retention. Occasionally, 'Urokolin' is useful to assist bladder emptying. Acute retention may be treated by intermittent or continuous catheterisation, urethral dilatation, or, if this proves unsuccessful, trans-urethral resection of the bladder neck using an infant resectoscope.

The infant metabolism is extremely labile. Even partial urinary obstruction— especially if accompanied by vomiting—can cause a rapid rise in the blood urea concentration, so this level needs to be checked periodically.

Infection must be recognised and treated, remembering that the infant may have a grave infection without any real symptoms. In choosing a suitable urinary antiseptic, it must be remembered that nalidixic acid and co-trimoxazole should be avoided in infancy.

Management in Early Childhood: the Pre-school Child

Periodic assessment

Parents and nursing staff should keep a constant watch on the efficacy of bladder emptying and signs of possible infection. They must be taught what to look out for. When there have been obstructive symptoms in infancy, the IVP should be repeated in six months, since gross hydronephrosis can develop quickly (Fig. 11.3). In all other cases, the IVP should be performed annually. It is particularly important to forestall serious deterioration, as renal cortical damage is irreversible. Severe acute urinary infections may upset the balance of hydrocephalus, and, by sweating and vomiting, cause biochemical disturbance requiring hospital admission. On such occasions, the opportunity should be taken to investigate and regulate the urinary tract and to give the parents an intensive course in bladder management. At this stage a micturating cysto-urethrogram is valuable and occasionally bladder neck resection, or sphincterotomy is shown to be necessary.

Even in cases with an apparently normal central nervous system, attainment of continence may be delayed. Little is to be gained from attempts to toilet train before the age of three or four years. It is worthwhile, however, asking the mother to note hopeful signs, such as a napkin remaining dry for two hours after expression. In this age group it is particularly important to ensure that fluid intake is not being curtailed, either from natural reluctance to drink or from the mother's unwise attempts to keep the child dry.

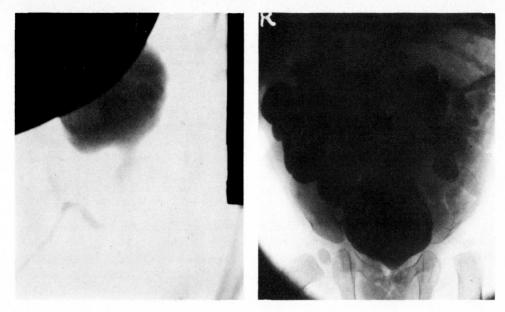

Fig. 11.2 (*left*). Micturating cystogram. Expressible bladder. Pressure from a lead glove (*above left*) starts urine flowing but there is considerable residual urine.
Fig. 11.3 (*right*). Intravenous pyelogram. Nine-month-old patient. The upper tract was undilated at birth.

Though it is debatable whether urinary diversion is justified for purely social reasons below school age (but see p. 000), there is no doubt that it may become necessary for surgical reasons if renal damage cannot be avoided by conservative means.

Many spina bifida children need orthopaedic operations in the first five years of life. It is essential that there should be a co-ordinated plan of action. Operation sites round the hip may become contaminated by urine, so it is better to avoid an abdominal diversion until hip surgery is completed. A patient in a hip spica presents problems for urine collection. Where regular expression has been practiced, it is often possible to continue this by cutting the plaster away round the pubic area. In other cases, an indwelling Foley catheter provides the best drainage. Fluid intake must be high and a prophylactic urinary antiseptic may be advisable.

Some children have renal damage by this age and are liable to recurrent infections, each of which must be supposed to cause further damage. They should be kept on a maintenance dose of one of the safer urinary antiseptics such as sulphadimidine, co-trimoxazole or nitrofurantoin.

The appropriate precautions should be observed, and the more dangerous antibiotics reserved for super-infections causing serious symptoms.

Management of Older Children and Adults

Re-examination of the urinary tract should be continued at intervals not longer than six months in all cases with a significant neurological deficit, even for those who have achieved continence, for these may have continuing silent pyelo-nephritis.

Most patients should have an annual IVP. If the anatomy of the collecting system remains near-normal, and the renal cortices do not become scarred and thinned, there is little danger of renal failure. If deterioration is noticed, it is important to test the urine regularly, perform renal function tests, measure the blood pressure and x-ray the hands and wrists for renal rickets. A habit of high fluid intake should be established in such patients. From this time on it must be the aim to establish a stable urinary tract which does not deteriorate, and a hygienic method of passing and collecting urine in a way that will give independence from the care of other people. Renal damage or mental and physical disability will often frustrate these aims, and sometimes all that can be done is to try to forestall further decline.

Monitoring of Progress

Urine testing

Whether the urine is required for biochemical analysis, cell count or culture, it is important that the specimen be as clean as possible. Bacterial contamination rapidly reduces the value of all forms of testing, so the specimen should be examined within 30 minutes of collection or else refrigerated.

A clean catch specimen (preferably mid-stream) obtained after thorough cleansing of the parts and drying to remove residual antiseptic is suitable for older children or adults. Those with no voluntary micturition may have manual expression. Babies or those with involuntary emptying may have Paul's tubing or a sterile disposable adhesive plastic bag (U-Bag, Hollister Co.) fitted. The only way to ensure a completely uncontaminated specimen is by suprapubic puncture (Pryles et al. 1959). This is a simple and safe procedure provided that it is performed only when the bladder is palpable above the pubes, as is usually the case in infancy. There should seldom be any need to pass a urethral catheter solely to collect a specimen. Specimens taken from an ileostomy bag or penile urinal are useless unless the parts are cleaned and a new bag fitted. The best method of collection from an ileal loop is by catheter, but Smith (1972b) has shown that a single catheter picks up organisms on its way in, and recommends first passing a large catheter and threading a finer one down its lumen into the depths of the loop. The additional advantage of catheterising a loop is that it reveals excessive capacity usually caused by stomal obstruction.

For routine screening, especially if facilities for collection are unsatisfactory, there is much to recommend a dip-strip method. Dry culture medium on a plastic strip (innoculated by holding in the stream of urine or dipping into a freshly passed specimen) is sealed in a plastic envelope and can then be incubated at room temperature or sent by post to the laboratory for sub-culture and sensitivity testing. An immediate indication as to whether the urine has been decomposed by organisms before leaving the body is obtained by a nitrite strip, responsive to most common organisms except Str. faecalis. The Microstix method (Ames Laboratory) combines these two facilities (Craig et al. 1973). Patients or their parents can take specimens in this way a few days before a clinic visit and send the strip to the laboratory. The result is then available at the time of follow-up. The only parameter not obtainable in this way is the cell count, which may be important to decide whether organisms are causing inflammation.

Excretion pyelogram

This is one of the most valuable tests since it demonstrates the anatomy of both upper and lower urinary tract, its patency and motility, and gives a reasonable indication of function. The bladder films taken after most of the dye has cleared the kidneys give a good idea of bladder capacity and the state of the urethral sphincters, and, after emptying, of residual urine and ureteric reflux (Fig. 11.4).

The neonatal series is used as a baseline for examinations repeated at intervals of six to 24 months, depending on conditions. The intravenous route should nearly always be available, and discomfort can often be avoided by finding a vein in the insensitive lower limb.

As these patients are often constipated, special care is needed in preparation of the bowel before x-ray. It is often impossible to clear the field completely, and if the control film shows the kidneys to be obscured, the 'Pepsicolagram' technique may be used, distending the stomach with gas by giving a drink of soda water or injecting air down a feeding tube (Fig. 11.5).

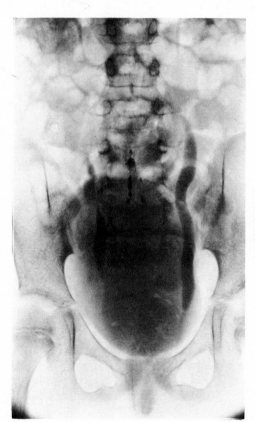

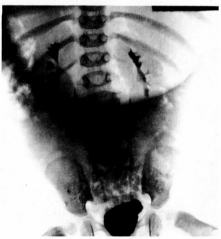

Fig. 11.4 (*left*). Intravenous pyelogram. End of excretory phase. After micturition with manual expression there is still gross residual in a flaccid bladder. Urine has refluxed into both ureters.
Fig. 11.5 (*below*). 'Pepsicolagram.' The pelvi-calyceal pattern and renal outlines are seen more clearly through the stomach bubble.

Micturating cystogram

This is necessary in cases where the IVP fails to give sufficient information about the filling and emptying of the bladder to permit a decision concerning control of continence, relief of outflow obstruction or ureteric reflux. Filling the bladder with medium through a urethral catheter carries a high risk of infection, and a catheter is also liable to disturb the action of the sphincter if left in place too long. Supra-pubic puncture is therefore preferable, but, if it is impossible, the finest possible urethral catheter should be used. Films taken with the bladder distended give a good idea of capacity, the presence of trabeculation, diverticula or saccules, and whether ureteric reflux occurs (Fig. 11.6). A completely flaccid external sphincter makes filling impossible; dye runs out of the bladder as fast as it is injected (Fig. 11.7). If the bladder neck is relaxed, urine fills the posterior urethra, being held up by an active external sphincter (Fig. 11.8).

Cystometrogram

A standardised technique for this procedure (Cooper 1968) has made it a valuable research tool, but the information it yields can often be deduced from clinical observation and the foregoing investigations. It is not needed in every case, therefore, but can be very helpful. Most cases fall into a definite category (Figs. 11.9), although a few defy classification.

When taking pressures it is important to isolate intrinsic bladder contractions from total intra-vesical pressure. This is found by subtracting intra-abdominal pressure (most conveniently recorded by a rectal pressure probe) from the pressure measured with an intravesical probe.

In difficult cases, synchronised pressure, flow and x-ray recordings are valuable (Bates and Corney 1971).

Urethral pressure profile

Lateral pressure exerted by the wall of the urethra as a catheter is withdrawn gives useful information about outflow resistance at the bladder neck and external sphincter, and supplements the cysto-urethrogram (Brown and Wickham 1969, Edwards and Malvern 1972*b*). Pre-and post-operative tracings are particularly useful in demonstrating the effect of dilatation, bladder neck resection, sphincterotomy or pudendal neurectomy (Fig. 11.10).

Electromyogram

A fine concentric needle electrode thrust into the external sphincter or transverse perineal muscle records action potentials, but makes no distinction between voluntary and involuntary activity. There is, therefore, seldom any useful application of the method during initial assessment, but recording of the EMG in external sphincter gives evidence of the success of denervation by pudendal neurectomy or subarachnoid injections of phenol.

Radio-isotope studies

Radio-isotope studies may be useful in patients with failing kidneys, unsuccessful IVP, or those prohibited by iodine allergy. The presence and anatomy of functional renal tissue on each side is demonstrated by a *renal scan,* while function in each kidney is assessed by plotting the time-course of radio-activity using a pair of accurately placed scintillation counters (*radio-isotope renogram*) (Cudmore and Zachary 1970).

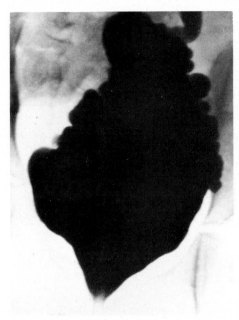

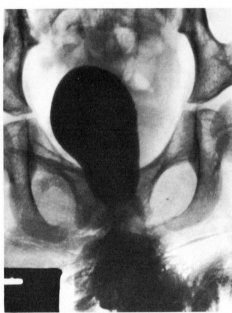

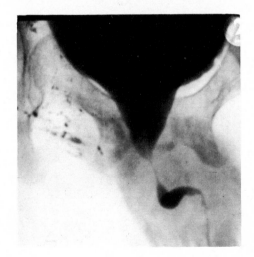

Fig. 11.6 (*above left*). Micturating cystogram. Flaccid bladder, towering, trabeculated and refluxing.

Fig. 11.7 (*above right*). Micturating cystogram. Flaccid sphincters. Dye runs out of the bladder around the urethral catheter.

Fig. 11.8 (*right*). Micturating cystogram. Open posterior urethra. Active external sphincter.

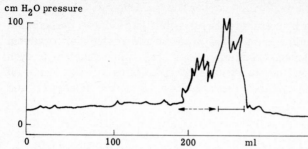

Fig. 11.9. Cystometrograms. Normal bladder pattern. Detrusor contractions are inhibited and pressure remains low until emptying is desired and initiated by straining.

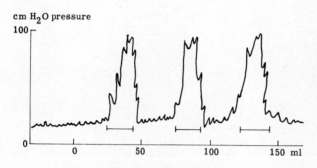

Reflex bladder (Group I). Uninhibited pressure waves give rise to involuntary voiding of small amounts. The external sphincter fails to relax so high intravesical pressure does not empty the bladder completely.

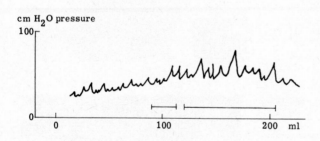

Partially denervated bladder (Group II). Resting pressure rises steadily until outflow resistance is overcome, when dribbling commences. Bladder contractions continuous but aimless. The bladder is expressible.

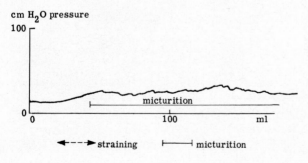

Completely denervated bladder and sphincter (Group III). Pressure never rises because urine trickles past the patulous sphincter and the bladder cannot be filled.

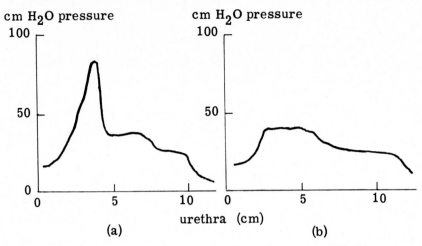

Fig. 11.10. Urethral pressure profile (a) before and (b) after transurethral sphincterotomy.

Renal function tests

It is not necessary to perform specific renal function tests on those patients with consistently normal urine and normal or near-normal IVP, but in those where successive examinations show increasing hydronephrosis, pyelonephritic scarring or loss of renal cortex, renal failure should be anticipated. Regular serum urea or creatinine levels should be performed, though they may be misleadingly normal in a patient who is close to renal failure. More warning is given by the creatinine clearance test, though this too is subject to error. The degree of opacification seen on IVP films gives a rough guide, especially of differences between the two kidneys. The same information is gained somewhat more accurately by the radio-isotope renogram.

Blood pressure

Readings of blood pressure are not a routine in most paediatric clinics, and it is not easy to make an accurate measurement in young children. Hypertension due to renal failure is unlikely to occur in the first decade of life, but it should be watched for after this in those with x-ray evidence of a deteriorating renal tract.

Promotion of Drainage

Urinary throughput is of prime importance in maintenance of renal function and prevention of infection. Copious fluid intake at frequent intervals must become a habit and in childhood be supervised by parents and teachers, especially during periods of abnormal extra-renal fluid loss caused by febrile illness or hot weather.

Though there is a higher than normal incidence of upper renal tract abnormality in spina bifida, the vast majority of obstructions are below the bladder. However, ineffectual pelvic and ureteric contractions and atony of the bladder lead to stagnation even in the absence of obstruction, so that drainage often has to be encouraged.

137

Manual expression

This is often called the Credé manoeuvre, but in fact Credé's original description was of a method of emptying the uterus. About 40 per cent of spina bifida patients have an expressible bladder, but the amount of urine obtained depends upon the relative activity of detrusor and sphincter. Some have a high bladder capacity and considerable sphincter resistance. In these, useful quantities of urine may be expressed, but there will also be considerable residual. At the other end of the scale, the detrusor has some tone but the sphincter none, so that posture and intra-abdominal pressure, as well as bladder tone, will keep the bladder almost empty, and there will be little urine to express.

Those with upper motor neurone or mixed lesions can sometimes be expressed but suffer from unco-ordinated contraction of the external sphincter, which may be brought on by voluntary or reflex activity in other parts of the body. Often, if the patient can be encouraged to relax generally, urine will flow but will stop abruptly if he strains, cries or moves the trunk.

Technique   In the infant or young child it is easier for the mother or nurse to express the bladder with the patient lying supine on a firm mattress. As the child becomes bigger and heavier this becomes more inconvenient, and a squatting posture on a commode or toilet seat is more desirable. It is to be hoped that eventually he will have the manual strength to express himself, aided by thigh flexion.

Each individual bladder behaves differently, so it is necessary for a suitable personal technique to be developed. Sometimes a firm, pear-shaped mass can be felt rising from the pelvis. This can be grasped between fingers and thumb and pushed bodily down and back in the direction of the perineum. Alternatively, the flat of the hand can be used to apply pressure to the lower abdomen. It is important not to exert pressure too low down or the fundus of the bladder may escape upwards. Some parents are tempted to use excessive pressure which, besides being painful and self-defeating, may be dangerous. One inventive but misguided father even prepared designs for a system of levers like a giant wine-press. It is more rewarding to exercise gentleness and patience with intermittent pressure while watching for results. Some of the most successful expressions are in fact triggering of reflex emptying by stroking, tapping or lightly pressing the lower abdomen, while such bladders will be impossible to empty if roughly handled, because the external sphincter goes into spasm.

There are three reasons why a bladder may not be expressible:
(1) it is normally innervated;
(2) the sphincter is in spasm;
(3) it is empty.

If a bladder is regularly expressible, it is usually desirable to establish a routine by the clock, related to the child's age and tendency to infection. The only reservation is the presence of vesico-ureteric reflux. Though some authors (Pekarovič *et al.* 1970) make this a definite contra-indication, it would seem sensible to weigh up each case on its merits. If reflux is accompanied by atony and there is no outlet obstruction, there would seem more to be gained than lost by regular expression. Sometimes, when reflux is unilateral, it may be helpful to press with one hand over the affected kidney while expressing the bladder with the other.

Cholinergic drugs

Those patients in whom manual expression leaves an unacceptably large residual may be helped to empty their bladders more completely by the use of a cholinergic drug. Urocholine is probably the most suitable (Ardran *et al.* 1967).

Bladder neck procedures

A decade ago, bladder neck hypertrophy was often blamed for outflow obstruction. Most surgeons agreed that open procedures such as Y-V plasty were less suitable for neuropathic bladders than trans-urethral resection. (Eckstein 1968, Nash 1970). An overactive, obstructed bladder may be expected to develop hypertrophy around the bladder neck, but it is doubtful whether this is the cause of obstruction. In recent years, attention has been focussed on the external sphincter, and it seems likely that it is usually an overactive, decentralised, external sphincter that is responsible for poor emptying of the bladder. However, a deep suprasphincteric cut with a diathermy loop may, in females, produce a permanent urethro-vaginal fistula which effectively relieves obstruction, though removing any chance of toilet training.

Destruction of external sphincter

Occasionally, in the newborn, it may be sufficient to *dilate* the urethra with sounds to overcome retention. Usually, however, it is necessary to cut the sphincter, preferably by diathermy. In male infants, a perineal urethrotomy may be needed in order to pass even the smallest infant resectoscope (about 13 Charrière gauge). Disappointing results may be due to insufficiently deep cuts. Lendon and Zachary (1974) studied cadaveric material and concluded that lateral cuts of up to 4.25cm depth would be required to divide the muscle completely. Paradoxically, an adequate *sphincterotomy* may relieve obstruction, and, by making manual expression more efficient, improve continence (Malament 1972, Nanninga *et al.* 1974) *Pudendal neurectomy,* by cutting the anterior division of both pudendal nerves, should completely relax the external urethral sphincter while leaving the anal sphincter intact. It is not an easy operation in a small, fat child, and failure is not uncommon (Stark 1968*a*, Engel and Schirmer 1974). A more reliable method is the repeated injection of *phenol* into the terminal sub-arachnoid space, but is justified only if the anal sphincter can also be sacrificed (Merrill and Conway 1974).

Catheterisation

Intermittent catheterisation may be necessary in the neonatal period for acute retention, and should be followed by urethral dilatation or sphincterotomy. An indwelling Foley catheter is often useful during orthopaedic operations on spine or hip where manual expression may be difficult. Long-term Foley catheterisation has been used mainly for continence (see p. 146), but there are occasions when the balance of the factors involved would tip in favour of the improved drainage rather than the disadvantage of a foreign body.

Ureteric reimplant

After outflow obstruction has been relieved, uretero-vesical reflux often persists, so that even if the bladder is efficiently emptied, stagnation and infection will continue. Reflux-preventing operations (Politano and Leadbetter 1958, Paquin 1959) would seem unlikely (on theoretical grounds) to succeed in the flaccid neuropathic bladder, since competence depends on an actively contracting detrusor; nor are they likely to stop reflux in a thick-walled unco-ordinated bladder. Johnston, however, has had at least short-term success (Thomas *et al.* 1975). If careful selection is made, a few cases may be found in which reflux seems to be due to the presence of a juxta-ureteric diverticulum, and, in these cases, reimplantation is justified.

Long-term follow-up of the urinary tract in spina bifida (Rickham 1964, Smith 1972*a*) shows that deterioration cannot be halted unless it is tackled at an early stage. Therefore, unless conservative methods of promoting drainage and controlling infection are effective immediately, permanent diversion away from the bladder should not be delayed.

Cutaneous Ureterostomy

When the bladder is patulous, the renal pelves dilated, and the ureters redundant and tortuous, improvement of the bladder outlet cannot be expected to relieve stasis. A temporary loop-ureterostomy in one or both flanks (Fig. 11.11*a*) may allow hydronephrosis to subside within a few months. Bilateral loop-ureterostomies are not a satisfactory permanent arrangement because of the difficulty of collection from separate stomata, and so, if continuity cannot be safely restored, they should be converted to a more satisfactory form of diversion with a single stoma.

End ureterostomies are suitable for permanent use, provided that at least one ureter is long enough to reach the optimum position on the abdominal wall for fitting an appliance, allowing enough length to fashion an everted stoma. If the other ureter is of normal length and diameter it can be joined in Y-formation to the larger one (Fig. 11.11*b*). It should be remembered, however, that in other circumstances, notably a naturally bifid collecting system, a Y-formation may be an inefficient arrangement (the 'yo-yo' effect). Usually, both ureters can be brought to the surface together as a double-barrelled stoma (Fig. 11.11*c*). In cases where the ureters are not quite long enough, a short stomal segment of colon can be added (Nixon and Kapila 1968) (Fig. 11.11*d*).

Ileal loop

First, it is necessary to condemn the use of the term 'ileal bladder', since this implies a container which fills and empties, and this is definitely not the intention. Many laymen—and even doctors—have been misled into the belief that such a diversion is meant to retain urine. In fact, of course, it will only do so if there is stomal obstruction—and this is a certain recipe for disastrous infection. An efficient ileal loop or, alternatively, colonic loop (Mogg 1967) is generally regarded as the most effective form of permanent drainage for a neuropathic urinary tract. Operative techniques are fully described elsewhere (Bricker 1950, Nash 1956, Rickham 1964, Smith 1965) and will not be elaborated, but for purposes of promoting drainage, certain rules need to be observed: redundant ureters should be shortened as much as possible; the loop of bowel should be as short as possible; a circle must be excised from all layers of the abdominal wall (Rickham 1964 uses a trephine to cut straight through); and a ring constriction must be avoided at the muco-cutaneous suture line. Smith (1965) makes a zig-zag scar by using a Z-incision through the skin. Efficient functioning is monitored by passage of a catheter (which should show no more than 10ml of urine in the loop), by regular IVPs, and, if there is suspicion of stomal obstruction or atony of the loop, by x-ray study of the dye-filled loop (Loopogram), (Fig. 11.12).

Choice of extra- or intra-peritoneal placement of the loop must be made after assessment of the relative advantages and risks. Rickham (1964) points out that a really short loop can be made only by running it directly from the sacral prominence to the anterior abdominal wall, and claims that the danger of intestinal obstruction is avoided by fixing the left margin of the mesentery to the posterior peritoneum.

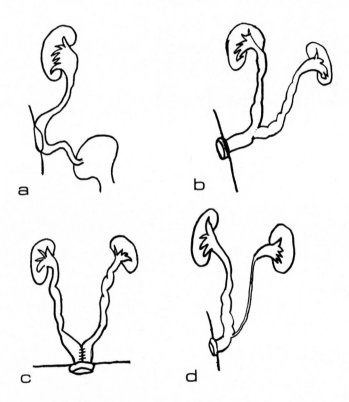

Fig. 11.11. Cutaneous ureterostomies.
(a) Temporary loop ureterostomy to improve drainage from the right pelvis.
(b) Stoma fashioned from the right ureter. The shorter left ureter anastomosed to it within the abdomen.
(c) Both ureters long enough to contribute to the stoma.
(d) Neither ureter quite long enough. Stoma fashioned from a short length of ileium.

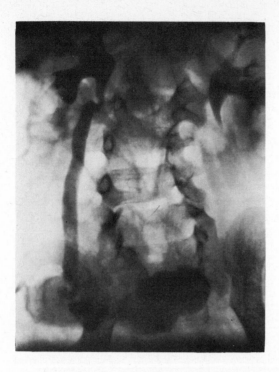

Fig. 11.12. Loopogram. Loop filled by a catheter in the stoma. Dye has refluxed into both ureters. Ten minutes after withdrawal of the catheter all contrast should have cleared the system.

A cogent argument in favour of a trans-peritoneal loop is that it is much easier to revise and shorten if it becomes redundant and urine stagnates (a residual in excess of 30ml). Pekarovič *et al.* (1968) showed that the intra-luminal pressure is often (but not always) higher in extra-peritoneal loops, sometimes exceeding the normal intra-ureteric pressure peaks. This could be a potent cause of the gradual deterioration that is sometimes seen in the absence of obstruction at the uretero-ileal anastomosis or the abdominal stoma.

In spite of meticulous techniques designed to avoid obstruction or stagnation, it cannot be denied that the long-term results of ileal loop diversion leave much to be desired. Many authors, presenting large series, have described late deterioration in the upper tract, most disturbingly in cases where it was normal before operation (Cook *et al.* 1968).

Care of the residual bladder

The bladder left isolated by a urinary diversion often becomes a reservoir of infection, especially if the outflow tract still offers some resistance. A copious, foul-smelling discharge appears intermittently, often wrongly diagnosed by the uninitiated as a vaginal discharge and inappropriately treated. Bladder washouts through a urethral catheter with 'Hibitane' 5 per cent usually clear up the trouble after a few weeks. Failing this, generous trans-urethral resection helps the bladder to remain empty, or, if these measures are not successful, it is occasionally necessary to perform cystectomy, a fairly simple operation in these patients.

Management of Infection

The main difficulty is in deciding what constitutes an infection in spina bifida. Difficulties in collection often make it uncertain whether there is a significant infection, and abnormalities of anatomy and hydrodynamics alter the significance of test results.

A culture of organisms is usually considered to indicate significant infection if it grows more than 10^5 colonies/ml, while one between 10^3 and 10^5 is borderline and should be repeated. Even a scanty growth from a percutaneous supra-public puncture specimen indicates infection. A mixed growth suggests a contaminated specimen, but may be of significance in chronic infection or the presence of a loop.

Pyuria may be considered significant if over 10 cells/cm are found in a fresh specimen.

Four situations commonly arise:—

(1) *A patient presents with a febrile illness, perhaps also with symptoms suggestive of raised intra-cranial pressure. The urine shows a significant number of cells and organisms. Is urinary infection the cause of the illness?*

In such a case, if no other infective focus can be found by clinical or laboratory investigation, it is appropriate to treat with a course of a urinary antiseptic to which the urinary organisms prove sensitive.

(2) *Significant growth is found on routine culture in a symptomless patient with a reasonably normal upper tract. Should treatment be given?*

Routine tests at special schools, clinics, *etc.* are often carried out by very unsatisfactory methods, and the significance of test results is often very doubtful. Even after techniques are tightened up, the importance of finding organisms in a paralysed bladder or loop is uncertain. Nicholas (unpublished data), using Fairley's technique on these bladders (Fairley *et al.* 1967), found that, after bladder washout, the fresh urine coming down from the kidneys under diuresis was clear, suggesting that the bacteruria was confined to the bladder. It is therefore probably justified to take no action. Certainly, the temptation to treat resistant organisms with exotic antibiotics should be resisted.

(3) *A patient is subject to recurrent symptomatic urinary infections. Should antibiotics be confined to each attack or should he be kept on a maintenance dose?*

Each case must be assessed on its own merits, but frequent attacks, especially if accompanied by loin pain and with any deterioration in the x-ray appearances, make it justified to start long-term maintenance treatment. The most suitable drugs are sulphadimidine, co-trimoxazole, nitrofurantoin or nalidixic acid. In mild cases it may be sufficient to give one small dose at bedtime (Bailey *et al.* 1971).

(4) *A patient with an irreversably damaged upper renal tract has urine which cannot be sterilised. Resident organisms, often Ps.pyocyanea or B.proteus, are sensitive only to potentially dangerous antibiotics. Should the infection be treated while the patient is symptom-free?*

In such patients one should accept the inevitable and continue with maintenance drugs only. Bladder washouts or irrigation of the loop or ureterostomies with

'Noxyflex', 2.5 per cent or 'Hibitane', 5 per cent are often helpful and, of course attention must be paid to urinary throughput.

Continence

The attainment of urinary continence begins to concern the parents by the time the child reaches the age of about two years, though few can expect much control before four years. However, it is often possible to predict the likely outcome before then by study of the bladder pattern. Decisions about management are closely linked to maintenance of drainage and prevention of infection.

Napkins

There is nothing unusual or difficult about keeping infants or young children in napkins, but as they become older, the amount of urine passed and the size of the patient make it increasingly difficult to find adequate equipment, and the cost of disposable pads becomes considerable.

A few patients, by virtue of severe mental handicap or gross physical deformity, cannot be treated in any other way and it becomes essential to find the most suitable equipment and exercise meticulous care to keep the napkin area clean.

Because of the volume of urine produced, it is usually necessary to cover the napkins with plastic pants. These need to be carefully chosen to avoid tight edges cutting into anaesthetic skin, or, on the other hand, being so loose that urine leaks out. Disposable plastic sheets which tie at the hips ('Sofdown') or plastic pants with an inner pouch for the disposable absorbent pad ('Kanga') are usually suitable. Frequent changing is essential to avoid ulceration of buttocks or genitalia. It may be necessary to expose the skin under a bed cradle from time to time.

Time-training

An expressible bladder should be expressed from infancy to avoid urinary stasis. When the child is about two years old, parents and nurses can begin to adjust the time intervals for expression with a view to training, starting with an interval of one and a half hours and noting if the napkin is dry when next removed. With success, the intervals can be increased to two, and then three, hours, varying from time to time with varying activities and fluid intake, but never beyond three hours, for fear of infection. About 30 to 50 per cent of children can reach an acceptable degree of continence in this way by the age of four or five years (Forrest 1974, Nergårdh *et al.* 1974).

Those with a reflex bladder are very unpredictable. They are unlikely to be expressible unless external pressure can be made to trigger off micturition. Attempts at expression are more likely to cause tightening of the sphincter.

Prospects of success are affected by the sensory supply. A few patients have something approaching the normal sensation of fullness, others have a painful sensation when the bladder becomes overfull. Many can tell when urine begins to pass down the urethra, but most know nothing until it wets the skin above the sensory level. Surprisingly, a few patients quite suddenly develop definite sensation at the age of five years or more, which helps them to become aware of the need to pass urine.

Some mothers begin to think that their child is wet because of laziness, not

144

realising that sensory appreciation of the state of the bladder is missing, and that to keep constantly dry the spina bifida child must apply more concentration than a normal child.

Toilet training often depends on close observation of the child's pattern of micturition and detailed instruction to mother, nurses and teachers so that everybody knows what can be expected and the most satisfactory way of achieving maximum control. A period of residential training in a unit equipped with all facilities for investigation, and nursing staff experienced in the problems involved, can often turn the scales in favour of continence.

Many children who have achieved some control by the age of five years in the security of their own home may relapse when faced with the increasing demands and activities of school life. They must be told to resist the temptation to reduce fluid intake in an attempt to keep dry.

Successful control of urine is prejudiced by a loaded rectum. In some cases, manual expression empties the rectum as well as the bladder, but the bowel usually needs separate management (see p. 152).

When the child is young, manual expression is usually easier when he is lying supine. Later, it is more convenient if he can be sat on a commode or normal toilet seat. This is not always easy because of the encumbrance of calipers. It is a great help if the bladder can be emptied without the calipers having to be removed.

Penile appliances

Males who cannot attain reliable control unaided can be kept dry with a penile urinal. This requires anatomical adequacy that is rarely achieved before the age of five years. Boys with fatty pubes or a small penis may be unsuitable until puberty or later. Rubber appliances are difficult to keep clean and may make the skin sore, but there is as yet no satisfactory appliance made wholly of plastic. It is desirable that there should be at least a semi-disposable plastic bag to be discarded every three days to keep down growth of organisms and minimise odour. There should be a non-return valve to keep urine away from the skin, and parents and others must understand that water will not flow uphill and that there must be no kinking or compression of the bag by clothing. The best arrangement is for the spout to protrude through a hole cut in the front of the underpants (swimming trunks rather than Y-fronts), and for the bag to hang free on the thigh or lie in a pocket stitched inside the trouser leg, with easy access to the drainage tap at the bottom.

For younger children, the pubic pressure urinal is usually best (Fig. 11.13), since the bag lies high enough to be worn under short trousers. It has the disadvantage of requiring tight groin straps, which may cut into the skin. Later, the penile spout urinal may be worn (Fig. 11.14); this is more dependent, but also requires groin straps. In older children and adults, the condom type of sheath is often preferable.

Ideally, there should be a fore-skin to protect the glans and external urethral meatus. If it is too redundant, partial circumcision is performed to get rid of ulceration. As with all appliances, expert advice on selection, fitting and maintenance is required. The author has found that with this service, nearly all boys can be kept dry. Others (Duthie and Stark 1974) have found the system less satisfactory.

145

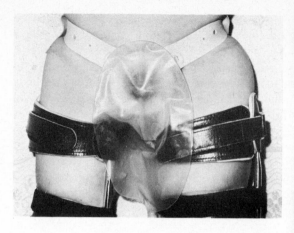

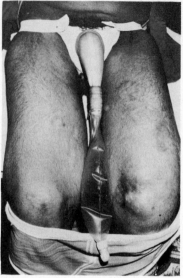

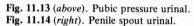

Fig. 11.13 (*above*). Pubic pressure urinal.
Fig. 11.14 (*right*). Penile spout urinal.

Many boys start to wear a urinal after failing to achieve toilet training. There is then a tendency to let urine dribble into it constantly and give up manual expression. An expressible bladder should still be expressed each time the bag is emptied, partly to avoid stagnation and partly to continue training. Some patients can stay reasonably dry without a bag and require to wear it only on special occasions.

Indwelling catheter

In the U.S., the indwelling catheter has been much used for draining the bladder in traumatic paraplegia (Comar 1967). In the U.K., however, the teaching of Guttmann (1954) has prevailed, and long-term catheterisation has been frowned upon (Eckstein 1974) on the grounds of supposedly inevitable infection. With the advent of non-irritating catheters of latex or 'Silastic', and of safe long-term urinary antiseptics, it now seems time for a reappraisal of the situation. Duthie and Stark (1974) and the author (Forrest 1974) have used catheters successfully in selected cases for long periods. Particularly noticeable has been the complete absence of the expected serious complications such as persistent cystitis, urethritis, calculus formation, contracted bladder, urethral stricture or upper tract deterioration. Patients treated continuously in this way for more than 10 years have shown no deterioration in the IVP.

The obvious candidates for this régime are those females whose grossly deformed trunk makes the application of an abdominal appliance impossible, or whose parents wish to avoid a major operation for a diversion of which the outcome is uncertain. Males who have found a penile urinal unsatisfactory may also be tried.

Not all patients prove suitable for catheter drainage. A completely flaccid sphincter will fail to grip the catheter sufficiently to prevent it leaking or even falling

146

out with the balloon still blown up. Previous operations to the sphincter may also spoil the field, especially if a vesico-vaginal fistula has been produced.

Short-term catheterisation is sometimes undertaken to control infection arising from outflow obstruction or stasis. There is little doubt of its effectiveness in this way, and it is sometimes decided, for social reasons, to prolong its use. More experience is needed to show whether the presence of a catheter over a long period exacerbates or prevents recurrent infection, but it seems likely that it does more good than harm.

Insertion of the catheter must, of course, be performed with full aseptic precautions. It is certain that organisms quickly travel up the urethra alongside the catheter and establish themselves in the interstices of the latex tube. 'Silastic' is less receptive, however, and so these catheters can be left in place for four to six weeks without any recognisable urethral irritation, or, equally important, concretions on the balloon or in the lumen of the tube. The writer keeps all cases on maintenance doses of co-trimoxazole. Duthie and Stark (1974), however, use drugs only for manifest infections.

the smallest catheter that will prevent leakage is used—usually between 12 and 22 French gauge. The balloon is inflated as little as possible, often with only 3ml of fluid. As in any drainage system, attention to detail is needed to avoid kinking of the catheter or compression or overfilling of the bag. Dependent drainage is easier to achieve in a chair-bound patient than in an ambulant one. Once the method is established, it is usually possible to arrange the bag in the standing patient so that it lies no higher than the pelvis yet is hidden by short trousers or skirt.

One criticism of catheter drainage compared with an ileal loop is that the patient will always be dependent on others for help in changing catheters. Its great advantage is that it avoids a major operation and is not irreversible. Unlike an abdominal diversion, no harm is done if it proves unworkable.

Mechanical methods
(1) Prevention of dribbling after prostatectomy has often been achieved in elderly men by the use of the *penile clamp*. This method has been tried in the paraplegic, but with disastrous results because of the serious risk of ulceration of the insensitive skin.
(2) Vincent (1966) demonstrated the importance of elevation of the pelvic floor in controlling outflow from the bladder and has designed a balloon to be worn under the perineum to exert upward pressure. Again, there is an obvious risk to the anaesthetic skin, but the method does have logic in its favour.
(3) Working on the same principle, operations to raise the pelvic floor or increase the vesico-urethral angle (Millin and Read 1948) have been tried in spina bifida but without much success. The risk of increasing outflow resistance to the extent that it is too much for the poor tone of the detrusor is probably too great.
(4) Implanted synthetic materials have long attracted research, either for compressing or replacing the bladder (Friedman *et al.* 1964) or for replacing the external urethral sphincter (Bradley *et al.* 1971, Scott *et al.* 1974). Results so far suggest that it will be a long time before they are applicable to spina bifida patients. In the case of the bladder substitute, obvious difficulties arise in devising a system which will permit free flow from the kidneys and yet empty sufficiently completely to

147

avoid the evil effects of residual urine. In the case of sphincter replacement, the difficulty lies in the fact that the normal external sphincter is merely an ancillary aid to continence, and that compression of the urethra alone is not likely to be effective in the face of a permanently open and lowered bladder neck. The basic concept of such devices seems much too simplistic, ignoring the extreme subtlety of normal micturition. Timm and Bradley (1971) are working towards something more akin to the normal reflex by stimulating the detrusor to empty, replacing the sensory side of the reflex arc by placing a volume sensor on the bladder wall, and occluding the urethra by an inflatable plastic cuff, powered by metal bellows.

Electronic methods

Inspired by the success of cardiac pacemakers, work on incontinence devices was helped by the fund of basic experience in designing elctrodes and electronic circuits.

Unfortunately, however, stimulation of the bladder and its sphincters is a much more complex problem than cardiac pacemaking, and present devices fall far short of their aim to restore normal function.

Early attempts to stimulate the bladder directly were plagued by the problems of ionisation around the electrodes and by painful spread of electrical stimuli to other areas. When techniques were perfected in animals, it was found that the human bladder was more difficult to stimulate (Boyce *et al.* 1964, Ellis *et al.* 1964, Caldwell *et al.* 1965).

Considerable clinical experience of electronic stimulators has now been gained, particularly with the 'Mentor' stimulators. This device consists of specially designed electrodes, wound in a double helix and buried in folds on both sides of the bladder, which deliver bi-phasic impulses to the detrusor. Several excellent reviews describe its present status (Bradley *et al.* 1971, Edwards and Malvern 1972a, Merrill and Conway 1974, Halverstadt and Parry 1975).

There is difficulty in emptying the upper motor neurone lesion bladder because the reflex activity of the external sphincter and pelvic floor prevent outflow. Merrill and Conway (*op. cit.*) found that success could be achieved only by destroying pelvic floor spasm by repeated injections of phenol into the spinal sub-arachnoid space. Unlike striated muscle, the detrusor continues to respond to electrical stimulation after denervation, provided it has not been allowed to over-distend. However, a flaccid bladder is not like a normal one while at rest. While filling, it is like an elastic balloon and the natural configuration of the bladder neck is lost (Figs. 11.9c, 11.8).

Since it is not the external sphincter which is primarily responsible for continence, attempts at maintaining dryness by stimulating the sphincter are only slightly more physiological than replacement by a plastic cuff.

Patients with an upper motor neurone lesion have a sphincter that can be stimulated by implanted electrodes, but their trouble is usually more the inability to relax it. More important than the sphincter is the tightening of the levator ani which keeps the bladder neck elevated and prevents urine flowing. Caldwell (1963) places his electrodes in the levator ani rather than the external sphincter. If a way could be

148

found to inhibit, as well as stimulate, these muscles, we would be much nearer to success in the upper motor neurone lesion.

With a lower motor neurone lesion, the striated sphincter cannot be stimulated electrically unless its denervation and that of the pelvic floor is only partial. Those who have stimulated the sphincters and pelvic floor by anal plug, vaginal loop, or implanted pacemaker have had the greatest success in cases of mechanical rather than neurological damage to the muscles (Caldwell 1963). This is the type of case that can often be helped more simply by intensive perineal exercises.

Replacement of a functionless sphincter by a strip of intact gracilis muscle has been tried (Pickrell *et al.* 1956), but is not effective because voluntary control is required to keep it in tone. A pacemaker could be used to augment its activity (Nixon 1969).

A more promising line of approach in upper motor neurone lesions is to stimulate the sacral cord directly, which could perhaps produce a co-ordinated, reflex emptying of the bladder (Nashold *et al.* 1971, Grimes *et al.* 1973). In fact, this would seem more hopeful than Carlsson and Sundin's (1967) attempt to graft the second sacral roots to higher, intact ones.

Katona and Eckstein (1974) developed the entirely different concept of building up new micturition reflexes by passing electrical pulses into the bladder through a urethral catheter electrode for several hours each day. They seemed to have success in initiating normal emptying, but in a controlled trial (Eckstein, personal communication) results were disappointing. All of the apparently successfully trained patients relapsed. The same success could be achieved by daily catheterisation without switching on the current.

Work must clearly continue on electrical pacemaking, but it cannot yet be said to have widespread application to spina bifida. Edwards and Malvern (1972a) summed up the present situation by concluding that cases who might be helped by an electrical device are those most likely to achieve continence by other means.

Abdominal diversion

Many surgeons have concluded that an abdominal spout is the most satisfactory arrangement for incontinent females and have performed an operation at an early age, even in the absence of any surgical indication for improved drainage. Rickham (1964) is of the opinion that less psychological harm is done if the girl grows up with a stoma as part of her body image and cannot remember any other arrangement. While appreciating this philosophy, it should nevertheless be remembered that 20 per cent of children will achieve continence without diversion, and that, contrary to Lorber's (1971) report, even severely handicapped patients may become trained. Of the writer's patients with thoraco-lumbar lesions, 10 per cent have gained voluntary control.

An ileal loop diversion is a major procedure with a small mortality and a significant, immediate, and remote morbidity. There is no doubt that diversion occasionally causes dilatation in a previously normal upper renal tract. Seventy per cent of patients find it a satisfactory form of management, and, for some, it means the start of a new life; but the remainder, especially those of limited intelligence, continue

149

to have serious trouble with leaking bags that require changing several times a day, skin irritation, or stomal ulceration. A diversion is not advisable in cases with gross spinal deformity, where patient or parents are socially or mentally inadequate, or where a good appliance service is not available. Furthermore, once a loop has been formed, it is irreversible (Hendren 1973).

It is therefore important that each patient should be considered individually with regard to potential for toilet training, possibility of catheter drainage and likelihood of a successful and independent life with a diversion.

Points of technique were mentioned on p. 141, but for successful continence it is also necessary to make sure that the stoma is sited in the most favourable position. To this end, the appliance fitter should put on a suitable bag before operation, and, by submitting the patient to a full range of activities, find and mark the spot at which it most comfortably comes to rest over a smooth area of skin, well away from the rib margin and iliac crest. The laparotomy incision (whether transverse or vertical) should be made at least 5cm from the site of the stoma. A small sunken stoma is very unsatisfactory, and this often rules out cutaneous ureterostomies. Most surgeons fashion a stoma which is everted about 2.5cm, but Nash (1956) favours a much longer one which hangs over the flange into the bag, thus keeping urine away from the skin.

As the patient grows or becomes obese, it is sometimes necessary to revise the stoma or move it to a more suitable position on the abdominal wall.

Collecting-bags and their flanges were originally made of rubber and are still used by many patients. With the advent of satisfactory semi-disposable plastic bags, it has become easier to keep the collection of urine free from offensive odour and the stoma free from crusting. Plastic bags with a rubber flange (Fig. 11.15) are less convenient than wholly plastic ones (Fig. 11.16). On finding that a flange leaks, parents and nursing staff tend to add extra strips of adhesive round the periphery. It is better to review the whole appliance, especially looking at the technique of applying adhesive, and eliminating kinking or compression of the bag by clothing. It is not possible to standardise appliance techniques, since patients have widely differing needs. Each patient should have the appliance that is adapted best to the shape of the abdomen, quality of the skin and size of the stoma, as well as physical activity, type of calipers and clothing.

The most successful appliances may stay firm for many days, and some patients pride themselves on the length of time between changes. They should not, however, leave a bag on for more than three days, because infection builds up and may be transmitted to the loop urine.

Those with rubber bags should keep two, the spare one being scrubbed with soap and water or hung up filled with 'Hibitane', 5 per cent.

Patients with an awkwardly shaped abdomen who have found a conventional flange unsatisfactory may be able to manage with a semi-rigid plastic spout which takes the urine away form skin folds, rib margin or caliper bands and permits the bag to fill without pulling away from the body.

An intelligent patient can eventually learn complete independence, emptying the bag during the day, fitting a night bag to the bag's outlet at night (Fig. 11.17), and changing the bag every two or three days. A mirror on a flexible arm (Fig. 11.18) is helpful for this manoevre, since the patient lying supine tends to squirt urine over the prepared skin if he lifts his head to look at the stoma. After long practice, many learn to change their bag entirely by touch, without the help of a mirror.

Many patients as they grow older resent the interference with their privacy which incontinence may involve. Time spent in independence training is therefore well worth-while.

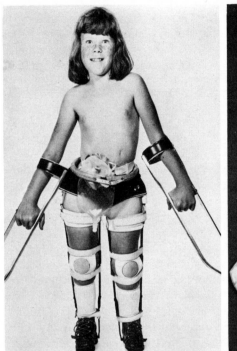

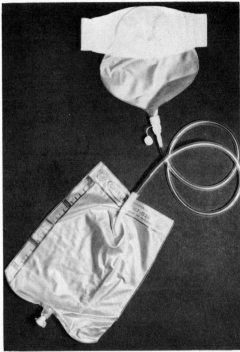

Fig. 11.15 (*above left*). Plastic semi-disposable ileal loop appliance.
Fig. 11.16 (*below left*). 'Newcastle' collection spout.
Fig. 11.17 (*above right*). Night bag attached to outlet of ileal loop bag.
Fig. 11.18 (*below right*). Mirror on flexible arm assisting self-application of bag.

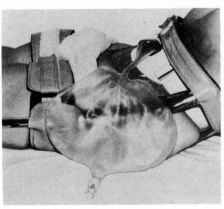

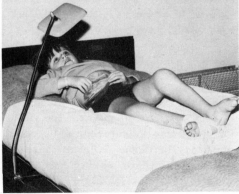

Care of the Bowel

The neurological state of the external anal sphincter is usually the same as that of the external urethral sphincter, since they have the same root innervation. Diagnosis of the state of the bowel is usually easier because the anal sphincter's activity is visible, and response to sensory stimulation can be seen and felt. The normal physiology is not so complex and the contents are more manageable.

Peristaltic activity is usually present in the terminal bowel, and expulsion of contents nearly always occurs spontaneously. There is, however, a tendency to constipation because of several factors, including lack of the sensory side of the reflex arc, dietary inadequacy, and general immobility of the patient. Once a state of constipation is established, there is a strong tendency towards rectal and colonic inertia.

Clinical types

As in the urinary tract, it is possible to distinguish different patterns of behaviour, though some individual cases defy classification.

Group I: The active sphincter of the upper motor neurone lesion. Stimulation of the peri-anal skin or insertion of a finger makes the sphincter contract vigorously. When the bowel contracts, the sphincter may relax to allow normal but involuntary evacuation. Some patients have overactivity of peristalsis and are troubled by frequent motions.

Group II: The sluggish sphincter of incomplete lower motor neurone paralysis. There is usually enough tone to contain the faeces (which are usually solid), and bowel motions occur at infrequent intervals. There may be some voluntary gripping, and even some response to electrical stimulation. The bowel contracts under the influence of aperients, or stretching by suppositories or enemata.

Group III: The sluggish sphincter of complete lower motor neurone paralysis. Often loosely closed while at rest, the sphincter dilates widely at the slightest stretching and remains gaping for several seconds before slowly shrinking down again to its resting position. There is no voluntary contraction or response to electrical stimulation. Fortunately, this type occurs in only five per cent of all cases.

Sensation is usually absent from the anal canal and peri-anal skin. Many patients get warning of the need to defaecate by the sensation of a full rectum. Others have no local sensation, but experience central or lower abdominal colicky pain when the bowel is ready to act.

Management

It is important to try to establish a regular bowel habit from infancy, and to avoid gross over-loading that could destroy any remaining stretch reflex. The motions should be formed and not too offensive, and this can best be achieved by attention to the diet. Some patients find that certain foods must be avoided because they cause disastrous diarrhoea. Additives containing roughage such as bran, or bulk such as methyl cellulose, are to be preferred to aperients such as 'Senokot', which are likely to cause unpleasant colic and act violently at unwelcome times.

152

A daily motion is not necessary. Many patients manage well by going on alternate days. On the other hand, too long an abstinence leads to overloading of the rectum with undesirable effects on bladder control and often overflow incontinence of faeces. As voluntary or reflex activity is established, many children learn to control their bowel motion either by sitting on a toilet seat or by abdominal pressure. Sometimes the bowel acts whenever the bladder is manually expressed.

Failing this form of control, it is most satisfactory to use a suppository. Either a simple bulk-forming preparation such as a glycerine suppository, or one with some pharmacological activity such as 'Dulcolax' may be successful. If this is inserted in the morning, a good motion 20 to 30 minutes later may allow the patient to remain clean at least until evening. A disposable enema has the same effect, but though more potent, may lead to troublesome faecal dribbling afterwards.

A few patients have no power to empty the rectum and require digital removal. Obviously, all these methods make the patient dependent on others, and, if possible, a regime which permits full independence should be found before adult life. In the first instance, however, it is most important to avoid colonic inertia and to try to find a way to avoid constant soiling. Most forms of urinary collection remain unsatisfactory until the bowels are properly managed, since bags and belts become contaminated.

A tiny minority of patients with lax sphincters have persistently loose motions. This usually makes control impossible, and can prevent any social integration. Regulation of diet, kaolin, or 'Lomotil' may be effective. The writer has had to resort to a permanent colostomy in less than one per cent of all cases. More often, a completely paralysed sphincter allows a hard pellet of faeces to escape without any effort or change in posture. This is not usually offensive, but in troublesome cases it would be worth considering insertion of a 'Silastic' Thiersch stitch (Hopkinson and Hardman 1973) to keep the orifice more firmly closed.

Prolapse

This is occasionally a problem from infancy, usually in cases where the whole pelvic floor is completely flaccid. Fortunately, it usually improves with age and is nearly always painless, although ulceration and bleeding of the rectal mucosa may be troublesome. Persistent cases can be treated by insertion of a Thiersch stitch. Of the rigid materials, mono-filament nylon is probably best, but it is seldom satisfactory since it has to be so tight to hold in the bowel that it prevents proper defaecation by the weakly propulsive rectal muscle, and may have to be removed. Hopkinson's method of using $\frac{1}{8}$ inch 'Silastic' rod shows promise. Intra-abdominal methods of fixation of the rectum are unlikely to succeed in these paraplegic patients.

Electrical stimulation

Group I and II sphincters that respond to stimulation rarely need help in maintaining continence: Group II sphincters are completely unresponsive.

Attempts to improve sphincter tone with an anal plug (Hopkinson and Lightwood 1967) must be avoided in patients with anaesthetic peri-anal skin because of the real risk of causing burns. The majority of patients with Group III sphincters have a low sacral lesion, sparing the adductor muscles. A gracilis sling would therefore be feasible. To obtain adequate muscle tone at all times, an implanted pacemaker is needed. Nixon (1969) has used this method with occasional success, but believes that further development is required before there is likely to be routine clinical application (personal communication 1975).

CHAPTER 12

General Paediatric Management

G. Stark

It is axiomatic that management of the child with multiple handicaps requires a multidisciplinary team. The paediatrician, especially if he has a neurological interest and training, can contribute to many aspects of management which have already been considered. He should be involved in neonatal assessment and the decision regarding operation. In some centres, the paediatric or paediatric neurology ward serves as the child's hospital base and the paediatrician is responsible for assessment of hydrocephalus and the electrophysiological studies of lower limbs and bladder which guide the surgeon's management. He is well qualified to treat infections of the CNS and urinary tract and to elucidate common diagnostic problems such as vomiting or convulsions. If, however, the responsibilities of each discipline are staked out in this way there is a danger that certain vital areas of management will fall into a no-man's land. If management is to be successful it must be problem-oriented rather than discipline-oriented.

To achieve this, one member of the team should have special responsibility for co-ordination of the hospital team and communication with parents and colleagues in the community. In particular, he must try to view the child—who is fragmented by specialised investigation—as an individual, and should assess the effect of disability on his everyday life and development. He must understand the impact of the handicapped child on the family and recognise their particular needs. He should recruit whatever help is necessary from other members of the team and from agencies outside the hospital to mitigate the more easily neglected social problems as well as the more obvious medical ones. He should have a relatively senior and permanent hospital appointment which will allow continuity of involvement over a period of years.

It is less important who accepts this rôle than that it should be well played. In most centres it falls to the paediatrician, but paediatric surgeons have also accepted the rôle with conspicuous success. It is not suggested that, in his guise as co-ordinator, the paediatrician should have a monopoly of communication, but simply that he should be identified by parents as a kind of medical ombudsman to whom they can, in the first instance, turn for help or advice at any stage in the child's management.

Serious shortcomings in the handling of parents and what they see as the real problems of the spina bifida child have been highlighted by several recent surveys (Hare *et al.* 1966, D'Arcy 1968, Freeston 1971, Walker *et al.* 1971, Richards and McIntosh 1973, Woodburn 1974). The paediatrician should be particularly conscious of these social, emotional and practical implications of spina bifida and in his attempt to understand them will find Mac Keith (1973) an invaluable guide to the feelings and behaviour of affected parents. These complex problems will now be considered in more detail and in a roughly chronological sequence.

Neonatal Period

In the flurry of preparation for transfer of the infant to the neonatal unit, the acute emotional plight of the mother is easily neglected (Walker *et al.* 1971). She is likely to have little knowledge of spina bifida and may be incapable of taking in a detailed account of all its attendant problems. She should, however, at least be told that her infant has a serious abnormality and requires full assessment to determine what, if anything, can be done to help. She should be told gently and as soon as possible after delivery, since unexplained silence or removal of her baby can only increase her distress. In the larger maternity units a paediatrician should be available to give this first explanation to both parents. Occasionally, however, the unenviable task falls to a nurse or midwife who may have little experience of spina bifida. In such circumstances, particular care must be taken neither to minimise the defect nor to destroy all hope. Woodburn (1974) found that what most mothers valued was 'an authoritative opinion given in a sympathetic framework'.

The mother should be allowed to take her baby in her arms and have a few minutes with her husband before they leave for the paediatric unit. In the state of helplessness, bewilderment and isolation which follows she needs particular care. She should be seen by the maternity hospital's medical social worker who can make contact with her counterpart in the children's hospital. It is not too early to involve the family doctor who must be kept informed of developments in the child's management. The mother should be allowed home as soon as she is able, but while in the maternity unit she requires meaningful reports on her child's progress and privacy in which to express her emotions.

In the paediatric unit the father can be given a clearer picture of the infant's condition and prospects. The information must, however, be given in simple language and the main elements repeated. If the child is considered to be a suitable candidate for operation, it is especially important that the father should understand what spina bifida involves before he signs an operation consent form. Parents must realise that even with operation the child may die and that the occasional untreated child will survive.

Where a selective policy is pursued, it is usual for the decision to operate to be made by the paediatrician and surgeons after thorough assessment of the child and in the light of their knowledge of the family background (Stark and Drummond 1973). The extent to which parents should be directly involved in making the decision is controversial. Ellis (1974) argues that, especially in borderline cases, they should be presented with the available options with the paediatrician acting as their adviser. Forrester (1968), on the other hand, considers that 'a half-anaesthetised mother and a distraught father are in no position to make rational decisions'. Others such as de Lange (1974) assert that the child's interest is paramount and that the doctor should act as advocate for the patient rather than the parents or society.

The parents of the infant not selected for surgical treatment need a great deal of support during the uncertain period preceding his death. A medical social worker can be of particular value in helping them come to terms with their feelings, not only of grief and guilt but often also of bitterness and hostility. They need specific reassurance that nothing they did or failed to do could have caused their child's condition. No less than the parents of the surgically treated child, they require reliable genetic counselling (see below).

The parents of the child selected for operation need detailed explanation of every step in management. Relatively simple procedures such as insertion of a valve to control hydrocephalus may have a profound impact on parents who have not been carefully prepared. Woodburn (1974) observed that 'the appearance of a small, shaved head with a large scar and black stitches was very distressing and deeply disturbing to many parents and the sight of the child post-operatively often the fact which brought home most painfully the realisation that the child was not normal'. It may be reassuring for parents at this stage to be shown a slightly older child who is progressing well following back repair and a CSF shunt.

The mother's anxiety about early surgical procedures may be matched only by her apprehension at the prospect of the child's discharge home. Unless she has been encouraged to handle, feed and get to know her baby from an early stage, she is likely to have little confidence in her ability to cope. Nevertheless, in her Sheffield survey, Freeston (1971) found that one third of mothers had never picked up their babies before the time of discharge. Young mothers particularly may welcome the opportunity to live in for a day or two before the child goes home, so that any practical problems may become apparent while help is readily available.

During the first admission, parents may be able to express their feelings and fears more freely to a medical social worker than to the paediatrician and surgeon responsible for the child's treatment. In such interviews, specific fears may come to light which can readily be allayed by medical staff. Before the child's discharge, the medical social worker should make contact with the appropriate community social worker.

As a result of the child's direct referral from the maternity hospital to the paediatric unit, there is a danger that the family doctor and local health visitor will be by-passed. A positive effort must, therefore, be made to involve them as soon as possible. In Edinburgh, the health visitor is invited to the paediatric ward where she can be briefed on day-to-day management and identified by parents as an extension of the hospital team. If the child is from a more remote area, one of the paediatric home nursing team can establish the link between hospital and community nursing services. In Cardiff, there is a liaison health visitor with a special interest in spina bifida who visits the child in hospital and discusses home management with the local health visitor (Bendix 1973).

A telephone call to the family doctor prior to discharge is more valuable than the detailed summary which arrives two or three weeks later. A copy of the discharge summary should automatically go to the appropriate department of community medicine.

When the child goes home, parents should be given an appointment for out-patient review within two weeks and should be reassured that in the meantime they need have no hesitation in telephoning the paediatrician, ward sister or medical social worker should any problems arise.

Genetic Counselling

Genetic counselling should be given to all parents who have had an infant

157

suffering from spina bifida cystica or anencephaly. The optimal time is within a month of the child's birth but not in the immediate newborn period as this is liable to increase the parents' feelings of confusion, guilt or inadequacy. There are strong arguments for genetic counselling being given by the paediatrician who must, of course, be well informed. He is likely to have established a good rapport with the parents; he will have a clear idea of the prognosis for their affected child and will be familiar with the local treatment policy. In view of evidence that genetic advice is frequently misunderstood (Walker *et al.* 1971, Woodburn 1974), the family doctor and social worker should know exactly what the parents have been told so that accurate information can be reinforced, as it must be, by repetition. Genetic factors in relationship to the epidemiology of spina bifida have already been summarised in Chapter 5.

It is estimated that the heritability of spina bifida in the United Kingdom is between 50 and 60 per cent (Carter 1974). The precise risk of recurrence of a neural tube defect in a family is influenced by the local incidence, but in the United Kingdom the risk is of the order of one in 20 when one child has been affected and one in eight after the birth of two affected children (Lorber 1965, Carter and Roberts 1967). The risk is further increased by consanguinity. If the previously affected child had spina bifida, approximately two thirds of the recurrence risk is for spina bifida and one third for anencephaly — and *vice versa*. It should be noted that the one-in-20 figure quoted includes not only the anencephalic likely to be stillborn and the infant with an extensive myelomeningocele who is unlikely to be selected for operation but also the infant with a closed myelomeningocele or simple meningocele with negligible neurological involvement. The risk of another child surviving with significant disability is, therefore, unlikely to be more than one in 50.

As well as information on the risks involved, parents can now be offered antenatal diagnosis in the next pregnancy which can be terminated if the fetus is affected. Detection in early pregnancy depends on the finding of elevated levels of alpha-fetoprotein in the amniotic fluid from pregnancies complicated by open myelo-meningocele or anencephaly (Brock and Sutcliffe 1972). The reliability with which these conditions can be predicted from amniocentesis at 14 to 16 weeks gestation has already been amply confirmed (Allan *et al.* 1973).

Although the risks of amniocentesis are small, it cannot be justified as a screening test in women who have no previous history of infants with neural tube defects. Maternal serum level of alpha-fetoprotein is, however, known to rise as an affected pregnancy advances and early results of its use between the 15th and 20th week of gestation are promising (Brock *et al.* 1974, Wald *et al.* 1974).

Provision of information on genetic risks and the possibility of antenatal diagnosis may not be enough. It may be necessary to ensure (by liaison with the family doctor) that practical contraceptive help is given. If a further pregnancy is contemplated, the importance of early booking at the maternity hospital should be emphasised and the indication for amniocentesis confirmed with the local obstetrician.

Hospital Follow-Up

The average child with spina bifida requires regular review by a paediatrician, paediatric surgeon (or neurosurgeon and urologist) and orthopaedic surgeon. Many patients also require the services of an ophthalmologist, plastic surgeon or other medical specialist. However necessary, hospital visits impose considerable stress on the family; they may involve many hours away from home and entail financial cost if, for example, the father has to take time off work. If the child has to be taken to a different hospital to see each specialist, not only is the number of hospital visits multiplied but confusion is likely to result for all concerned. Co-ordination can be improved if, as in Melbourne, a paediatrician accompanies the child and parents to each of the other specialist clinics (Field 1972).

In many British and American centres, however, an attempt has been made to integrate and simplify follow-up by establishing some kind of 'combined clinic' in one hospital, its precise form depending on local circumstances. If numbers are relatively small, as in Edinburgh, the child can be seen in the same room by the whole medical team, with ward sister, therapists and medical social worker in attendance. The paediatrician takes a developmental history and enquires about the child's and the parents' problems. As the child is examined by each specialist, the problems which have emerged can be discussed and a plan of management worked out. In this way, for example, the relative timing of hip surgery and urinary diversion can be settled and the siting of a stoma planned in relation to the child's future orthopaedic management. In order to achieve a relaxed, unhurried atmosphere conducive to satisfactory discussion of all the parents' worries and problems, a combined clinic of this kind can cope with no more than 10 patients per session.

An alternative arrangement is for the child and parents to remain in one room which is visited in turn by members of the team who later meet to discuss the patients they have seen (Hide and Semple 1970). While less overwhelming than the combined clinic, it has the disadvantage that a concerted plan for the next stage in management cannot be presented to parents when they are seen.

Neither of these systems is practicable if numbers are very large, as in Sheffield, where each doctor occupies a separate room and the child passes from one to the other as indicated.

If, as recommended, out-patient follow-up is concentrated in one hospital, it is easier to arrange for all relevant case notes and X-ray films to be available for the clinic.

Later Hospital Admissions

Hospital admission has a prominent and sometimes dominant place in the lives of spina bifida children and their families. Most children with myelomeningocele will have more than a dozen admissions in childhood and for a sizeable minority total hospital stay can be measured in years. With careful planning, much can be done to reduce the number and duration of hospital admissions and minimise the disturbance caused by those which are unavoidable.

Concentration of hospital care in one or two units means that the child will be in familiar surroundings and in the care of staff he knows. The concept of free visiting which is almost universal in children's hospitals and paediatric units is happily being increasingly accepted also in orthopaedic and neurosurgical units which admit children.

Even if it is unrestricted by the hospital, however, other factors may impose a limit on visiting. Foster (1973) has shown that the frequency of visiting is inversely related to distance from the regional centre. As distance from the centre increases, the cost and time involved increase rapidly. By public transport, for example, the time required for the round trip to the Royal Hospital for Sick Children (Edinburgh) from many Border towns is more than six hours and travel expenditure of between £5 to £10 per week is not unusual (Woodburn 1974). Although the importance of parental visiting is undisputed and was emphasised in the Platt Report in 1959, financial help is for the most part available only from charitable sources. The medical social worker associated with units admitting spina bifida children should be aware of local funds available for this purpose and there should be no hesitation in referring to her those parents who may be hesitant to mention the financial burden of visiting.

Difficulty in obtaining sufficient information about their child's condition ranks close to visiting as a source of concern during hospital admissions. The older child's need for explanation and reassurance is even more easily neglected, and it is most important, if the child is to return from theatre with his head shaved or his legs encased in plaster, that he has been prepared for this before the operation. Urinary diversion presents particular problems: one ward sister found it helpful to fit a miniature urinary diversion to the child's doll or a standard appliance to the child herself before operation. Parents with limited understanding of physiology require patient explanation and the opportunity of seeing another child with a diversion and of talking to his parents. Following any operation the parents must be given detailed instructions and practical demonstrations of management. For some parents, the handbooks published by the Spina Bifida Associations and other bodies prove helpful as a source of reference*: they are, however, no substitute for patient explanation by the clinician and nursing staff.

However much care is taken to maintain good communication with parents, hospital staff (who have to convey worrying information and are closely identified with the stresses of admission) must expect to encounter resentment and hostility at times. Such a reaction from parents has been aptly compared with the ancient Greek practice of killing the messenger who brought news of defeat in battle (Woodburn 1974).

Management at Home

Good management depends not only on skilful treatment of the child's medical problems but attention to those arising in everyday life. Although he cannot solve them directly, the paediatrician must be able to identify these problems and recruit appropriate help for the child and his family. In achieving this end, the value of home visits by hospital therapists and social workers cannot be exaggerated. They provide feedback to the hospital team and facilitate liaison with community therapists and social workers. Furthermore, advice and guidance provided at home, where mother and child are relaxed, is more likely to be effective than that given in the hospital setting, where, according to Walker et al. (1971), one mother said 'I can't hear what they are saying for nerves'.

*See list in Appendix II.

Practical Help

If secondary handicaps from environmental deprivation are to be avoided, the physically handicapped child must be helped to move around on his own and explore his surroundings. The spina bifida child who is unable to get about in the second year of life should have a small wheel-chair which he can propel about the house and a low trolley on which he can move around and play at floor level. A good example of the former is the 'Yorkhill' chair (Blockey 1971) and, of the latter, the 'Shasbah' trolley, both of which are now obtainable through the National Health Service. A light folding pushchair such as the 'Baby Buggy' makes it possible for a mother to take a pre-school child who is not yet walking on shopping expeditions and family outings. A larger version, the 'Buggy Major,' is available for the older child and can also be ordered through the N.H.S. by a hospital consultant. It is important that the parents and child understand that such aids are intended to widen the child's horizon at an early age and not as a substitute for independent walking. In appropriate cases, the mobility of the whole family can be increased by provision of a motor car which is possible through the Government's Family Fund.

The occupational therapist has a valuable rôle in assessing and helping with the difficulties of daily living such as feeding, dressing, toileting and play. She may find, however, that her advice is difficult to carry out in unsuitable housing conditions. (Woodburn (1974) found that two thirds of affected families in South-East Scotland were living in unsuitable housing conditions.) External and internal stairs are a common hindrance and may make the lavatory inaccessible to the patient. In some houses, doors are too narrow for wheel-chairs and in many there is a lack of storage space for walking aids, wheel-chairs and other impedimenta of the handicapped. Unsuitable housing not only limits the child's independence but increases the amount of lifting which the mother must do. Not infrequently, therefore, the most helpful single thing that can be done for the family of a spina bifida child is modification of the house or rehousing. Modification may be simply a matter of building a ramp up to the front door or may entail extending the house to provide a downstairs bedroom and lavatory. If rehousing is necessary *e.g.* in the case of a family living in high-rise flats, it should, if possible, be within reasonable distance of relatives. Recommendations for housing modification or transfer should be precise and based on reports by the occupational therapist and social worker. Local Authority Social Work and Housing Departments are, on the whole, sympathetic to such requests for help in improving housing conditions. The Family Fund may, however, be able to remedy deficiencies if assistance from other sources is not forthcoming.

The Parents' Associations have many schemes which provide practical help for families, including advice on equipment and appliances, babysitting services and assistance with holidays (for addresses see Appendix 2). Details of other sources of help for parents are included in the publications listed in Appendix 1.

Financial Support

The enormous financial cost of spina bifida to the community has been estimated by Lightowler (1971). The cost to individual families is also substantial (see Chapter 14). Extra expenditure is required on transport and on shoes and clothing which are

161

subjected to exceptional wear and tear. Parents may have to maintain a car and telephone which they would otherwise not require and the mother may be unable to work to supplement the family income. The Attendance Allowance which is intended to help towards expenses of this kind is not yet received by all parents who are entitled to it and must be brought to their attention. Additional financial assistance may be obtainable for specific requirements (*e.g.* shoes and clothing) from the Family Fund, Hospital Endowments, and other local charitable funds known to the medical social worker.

Emotional Support

With good medical management and provision of help with the innumerable practical problems of spina bifida, it should be possible to soften its emotional impact and prevent the state of helpless bewilderment encountered so often by Richards and McIntosh (1973). Inevitably, however, spina bifida will have some emotional and social repercussions which may require specific attention.

The effect of a spina bifida child on the parents' marital relationship, on siblings, and on the general emotional climate in the home is difficult to measure but has impressed several authors. In one of the few controlled studies, Tew *et al.* (1974) found that the divorce rate in South Wales for parents of a spina bifida child was more than twice that of control parents.

Many parents who may have difficulty in expressing their feelings and anxieties to one another or to the doctor treating their child need regular contact with someone with whom they can share them. This need is reflected in the high demand rate by parents for physiotherapy: in many cases it seems that the therapist is more important than her therapy. Continuous supportive counselling can perhaps best be provided by a local social worker who is in touch with medical aspects of the child's case through the medical social worker.

In some cases more formal group therapy sessions for parents have been organised and found rewarding (Linder 1970, Field 1972). Where the emotional impact on the patient or other children in the family is conspicuous, more specialised guidance from a department of child or family psychiatry is indicated.

Education

The pre-school spina bifida child has the same need as any other for group play which is so important for normal social maturation. He is, however, likely to need help in satisfying this need. Placing in a playgroup or nursery school from the age of three years is valuable for the child and, at the same time, affords the mother a regular period of relief. With adequate reassurance and practical guidance, *e.g.* from an occupational therapist, the staff of a normal play group can usually cope with a spina bifida child. In some areas, however, where facilities for nursery education are limited, small play groups for spina bifida and other handicapped children have been formed by Parents' Associations and other voluntary organisations.

Continuing developmental assessment is an essential part of the child's hospital follow-up, and this can be supplemented usefully by reports from occupational therapists, play group leaders and nursery school teachers. More formal psychometric assessment is, however, also desirable at the age of four years as the child approaches school age. While the assessment may be carried out by the clinical psychologist in hospital, the local educational psychologist has the advantage of close liaison with the education authority and school health service and may be able to test the child in more familiar surroundings.

Optimal school placing depends on good communication between the hospital team, psychologist, and school health service. It depends on the child's mobility, intelligence and sphincter control as well as geographical, social and other factors. In the last 25 years there has been a striking trend away from special schooling for the physically handicapped. In Scotland, in 1973, the number of children receiving special education on account of physical handicap was approximately one third of the figure for 1948; and, in 1974, only two thirds of places in residential schools for the physically handicapped were occupied (McHaffie 1974). Although there are considerable regional variations, a high proportion of spina bifida children are now attending normal schools.

Severe physical handicap and/or incontinence can, however, present over-whelming problems especially in antiquated school buildings with many stairs and primitive lavatory accommodation. In such circumstances, the child may be more appropriately placed in a day school for the physically handicapped, or, in the absence of local facilities, a residential school. In a small minority of patients, mental retardation will determine placing in a special school for the mentally handicapped or an occupation centre.

Full discussion with parents is essential and, if special schooling is recommended, they should be reassured that the placing is not final but will be reviewed and, if necessary, modified as the child's needs change.

Apart from the more obvious problems related to physical handicap. *i.e.* incontinence and frequent absence, other difficulties may become apparent in the school situation. As a result of hydrocephalus and CNS infection, more than two thirds of patients have neurological deficits in the upper limbs (Wallace 1973). Writing and other handwork may be impaired by inco-ordination, and particular difficulty may arise in the early stages of reading and spelling from visuo-spatial and other perceptual problems (Badell-Ribera *et al.* 1966, Miller and Sethi 1971). As a result, school performance may be poorer than the teacher at first expects from the child's relatively good verbal ability.

With sufficient preparation, explanation and support, teachers in normal schools are able to cope with quite severely handicapped children. The school medical officer should explain the necessary medical background to the teacher and a school visit by the occupational therapist can be of immense value in helping the teacher understand and overcome the practical difficulties that may arise in school and ensuring that the child is protected from physical hazards such as hot radiators.

Children in special schools are kept under close observation by the school doctor, who should be regarded as an extension of the hospital team. Good communication can be fostered by inviting the school doctor to the combined clinic or by periodic joint visits to special schools with the paediatrician. The School Health Service should receive regular hospital reports on affected children, whether in normal or special schools.

Adolescence

The emotional turbulence of adolescence is likely to be increased by anything which makes an individual 'different' at an age when the need to conform is paramount. As the normal adolescent is asserting his independence and becoming acutely aware of sexual feelings, his contemporary with spina bifida is becoming increasingly conscious of his dependence on parents and of his sexual limitations. Not surprisingly, the few studies which have been carried out on spina bifida in adolescence reveal a high incidence of social isolation and depression (Dorner 1973, 1974; Lorber and Schloss 1973). Adolescence is scarcely the best time, therefore, to hand the child's care over to a new team of doctors in another hospital. It is, however, an appropriate stage at which to establish contact with the local paraplegic service, which will later be responsible for follow-up. In centres where the same orthopaedic surgeon or neurosurgeon will be involved in care of adult spina bifida patients, the transition is particularly easy to achieve.

Employment

The problem of finding employment for school leavers with spina bifida has attracted attention only recently as the 'bulge' of patients treated in the early 1960s has approached school-leaving age. In the United Kingdom, the Department of Education publishes details of further education courses* and the Department of Employment is responsible for Youth Employment and Disablement Resettlement Services for the handicapped school leaver. Since, however, the problems of spina bifida are particularly complex, the question of vocational training and employment should not be left until the individual leaves school. During his last year, there should be discussions which may take the form of a case conference between the headmaster, educational psychologist, school medical officer and social worker, so that possible openings can be explored and discussed with the child and his parents before he leaves school. Parsons (1972) has shown that testing of aptitudes such as clerical skill, spatial ability, mechanical comprehension and manual dexterity can be helpful, at this stage, in selecting the most appropriate training and employment for individual patients. The proportion of leavers who are placed in open employment, sheltered employment and adult day centres will vary greatly from region to region, depending as it does on availability of employment and the severity of residual disability which, in turn, reflects the initial treatment policy.

*See Appendix I.

164

APPENDIX I

Publications for Parents

The following are published by the Association for Spina Bifida and Hydrocephalus, 30 Devonshire Street, London W1N 2EB:

Children with Spina Bifida at School, The Education, Training and Employment Committee of The Association for Spina Bifida and Hydrocephalus, 30p.

Clothing for the Spina Bifida Child, B. Webster, 15p.

Equipment and Aids to Mobility, O. R. Nettles, 25p.

The Nursery Years, M. Paull and S. Haskell, 15p.

Your Child with Hydrocephalus, J. Lorber, 15p.

Your Child with Spina Bifida, J. Lorber, 20p.

The Association also publishes a bi-monthly journal called 'Link' at 5p per copy or on annual subscription at 75p, post paid.

Other useful publications include:

The Challenge of Spina Bifida, A. Field, 40p, published by Heinemann Health Books, Tadworth, Surrey.

A Guide for Parents of Handicapped Children This is obtainable free of charge from the Scottish Education Department, Palmerston House, 6/7 Coates Place, Edinburgh.

Help for Handicapped People in Scotland Obtainable free of charge from Social Work Departments in Scotland.

The Spina Bifida Baby and *Growing up with Spina Bifida,* both available from the Scottish Spina Bifida Association (see Appendix II).

In the United States, the *Spina Bifida Association of America* publishes an extensive bibliography which is available, free of charge, from: The Library, Spina Bifida Association of America, P.O. Box G—1974, Elmhurst, Illinois 60126.

This bibliography lists books, pamphlets and articles covering all aspects of child care and development, including education, employment, laws and social services, schooling. It includes a list of children's fiction written especially about coping with mental and physical handicaps.

The societies listed in Appendix II also issue lists of their publications, on request.

APPENDIX II

Lists of Societies in the United Kingdom and North America

United Kingdom
Association for Spina Bifida and Hydrocephalus, 30 Devonshire Street, London W1N 2EB, England.
Disabled Living Foundation, Information Service for the Disabled, 346 Kensington High Street, London W.14., England.
The Family Fund, Joseph Rowntree Memorial Trust, Beverley House, Shipton Road, York YO3 6RB, England.
Scottish Spina Bifida Association, 7 South East Circus Place, Edinburgh 3, Scotland.
Scottish Council of Social Service, Information Service for the Disabled, 18/19 Claremont Crescent, Edinburgh, Scotland.

North America
Spina Bifida Association of America, P.O. Box 266, New Castle, Delaware 19720.
Institute of Rehabilitation Medicine, 400 East 34th Street, New York, N.Y. 10016.
Vocational Guidance and Rehabilitation Services, 2239 East 55th Street, Cleveland, Ohio 44103.
Association for the Aid of Crippled Children, 345 26th Street, New York, N.Y. 10017.
Committee for the Handicapped, People to People, 1146 16th Street NW, Washington D.C. 20036.
Co-ordinating Council for Handicapped Children, 407 South Dearborn Street, Chicago, Illinois 60605.

CHAPTER 13

Results of Treatment and Selection
of Type of Treatment

In the assessment of a newborn infant with spina bifida, and in discussing the likely prognosis with parents and relatives, some knowledge of the results of treatment is required. During the last 20 years the approach to the treatment of these infants has undergone some significant changes, and there are important differences between some of the centres principally concerned with the problem. It is now possible to assess the published surveys of results from a few of these centres in order to arrive at a policy which might prove generally acceptable.

Results of No Treatment—The Crude Survival

Prolonged survival of patients with quite extensive spina bifida lesions and hydrocephalus without any particular form of active treatment has been well described, and the report of the London Committee in 1885 is an outstanding record of this (see Chapter 1).

Laurence has provided the best analysis of the natural survival of patients with this condition from his detailed surveys in South Wales. 426 cases were identified as occurring between the years 1956 to 1962, and the occurrence rate of 4.1 per 1,000 total births has already been considered (see Chapter 5). By 1965 there were 67 survivors; 111 were stillborn, and 248 had died at various ages up to 10 years (Laurence 1966). From the results of a previous survey of a series selected by referral to hospital (Laurence 1964) the author inferred that deaths before the age of three months were from meningitis, and thereafter deaths in infancy and childhood were from hydrocephalus. Older children were more likely to die from renal complications.

In a later survey (Laurence and Tew 1966), 65 of the South Wales survivors were examined to ascertain the quality of their lives. 18 of these patients had meningoceles, all without accompanying hydrocephalus, and 13 of these patients were physically normal. The mean I.Q. was 94 in this group. Of the remaining 47 patients, 36 had myelomeningoceles and 11 had encephaloceles; 34 of these patients had major physical disability, 32 of them had suffered from hydrocephalus and the mean I.Q. was 86.

In summary, the survival rate of untreated patients with spina bifida aperta lesions is, therefore, 30 per cent at one year, 20 per cent at two years, and somewhat less thereafter. Only three and a half per cent of the whole series (including stillbirths) survive with normal or near-normal physical capacities and I.Q.s above 85.

Results of Treatment after Natural Selection—Delayed Operation

In the 1950s, interest in the surgical treatment of patients with spina bifida aperta lesions was renewed and by 1961, Guthkelch, in his 'Studies in Spina Bifida Cystica', was able to assess the results of a selective policy (Doran and Guthkelch

1961). The patients were referred to hospital around three months of age, and were operated upon if the neurological lesion was below T10 and the hydrocephalus not too advanced. There were 243 patients with myelomeningocele lesions (as opposed to those with simple meningoceles), of which 136 were operated upon and 107 were not. The assessment took place two and a half years after the last birth in the series and at this stage 70 per cent of the patients operated upon were surviving, compared with a survival rate of seven and a half per cent in those not operated upon.

The quality of survival was assessed in 55 myelomeningocele patients without hydrocephalus, and in 40 with hydrocephalus. There was mental impairment in 11 of the latter group, and putting the two groups together out of the total of 95 patients, there were 33 who were normal, 13 with minor disability, 29 with moderate disability and 20 with severe disability. In terms of percentages, this policy of operating on 60 per cent of those patients referred around the three-month stage produces a 43 per cent survival when assessed at two and a half years. The relationship of these results to the natural history of untreated spina bifida infants, as determined by Laurence's series, cannot be easily assessed, but from the life table study it might be assumed that those infants presenting at three months were the natural survivors, with the condition estimated at between 30 and 40 per cent. In this case, the delayed selection of 60 per cent of these for operation (out of which there is a 43 per cent survival at two and a half years) reduces the final incidence of the survivors to just over 10 per cent of the postulated original group, which is little different from the survival of the condition untreated. However, the quality of the survivors is clearly superior to that group defined in Laurence's series as having myelomeningoceles. A later analysis of the Manchester experience (Fernandez-Serrats et al. 1967) endeavoured to relate survival to the time of operation; there was a 68 per cent 12-month survival of those operated on before 48 hours, and a much lower percentage survival of those operated upon later. This general point, in addition to the observation that the quality of the survivors improved by rejecting the more impaired infants from surgical treatment, and that the occurrence of hydrocephalus is associated with a significant incidence of mental retardation, can all be gained from the Manchester experience. A policy which is partly dependent upon the time of referral, and partly upon neurological states which may have undergone post-natal deterioration, lacks the precision necessary for a more complete numerical evaluation of its effect upon the natural history of the condition.

The same reservations can be made over the more recently published Melbourne experience (Keys Smith and Durham Smith 1973), in which 295 patients born between 1961 and 1969 were studied. The age at which the infants were presented for treatment is not stated, but it is recorded that 79 of 295 patients received no active treatment, and of these 62 (78 per cent) had high lesions, by which is meant a neurological lesion above the lower lumbar segments (i.e. an infant with function in lumbar segments 1 and 2 would be regarded as having a high lesion). The other adverse criteria governing non-intervention were the early onset of hydrocephalus, infected myelomeningocele sacs, ventriculitis, or the presence of another life-threatening disease. Of the 214 infants who were surgically treated, 127 had the sac excised under 48 hours of age, and 87 over 48 hours, all of which indicates that the delayed referral of the infants must have constituted a significant factor in their selection for operation, and the results are likely to be different from those obtained by a policy based upon early referral. At the time of the survey, 55 per cent of those infants born between 1961 and 1965 were alive, and 61 per cent of those born between 1966 and 1969, and these are relatively high rates. The quality of survival of the 1961 to 1965 patients is nicely assessed by the determination that 39 per cent were at normal school, 59 per cent were at special school and two per cent were ineducable. 77 per cent had mental levels between high-normal and low-normal, and 23 per cent were mentally retarded, 31 per cent were ambulant without splints, and 69 per cent required short or long calipers or were not ambulant. Again, the same general points come out; the high lesions have a much higher mortality rate (whether treated or not) and a high incidence of hydrocephalus; furthermore, the early occurrence of hydrocephalus has also a high morbidity and mortality. In the hands of the Melbourne authors, whether the sac was excised before the age of 48 hours or not made no particular difference to the ultimate outcome in terms of infection and survival, but there was clearly a highly selective element influencing the decision to operate upon a child appearing after 48 hours of age.

Results of Unselected Treatment—Early Operation on All Patients

In 1963, Sharrard *et al.* published the results of a trial of immediate and delayed closures of spina bifida aperta lesions and produced evidence that improvement in muscle function followed early closure. This stimulated surgeons in many other centres to accept these children within a few hours of birth, and to close the back lesions within the first 48 hours. The effect of this early closure upon the neurological function of the lower limbs has now been analysed by a number of workers and can be related to the fuller understanding of the neuropathology of the spina bifida lesions (see below). There is now widespread recognition that early closure of the back lesion is not only the best means of preserving whatever neurological function the infant will ultimately be capable of but also achieves a radical reduction in the neonatal and infantile mortality by the prevention of infection entering through the open back lesion; this reduction in the mortality rate is the fundamental surgical principle behind early closure (Zachary 1966). The effect of this kind of policy upon the natural history of spina bifida aperta has been most clearly demonstrated in the experience from Liverpool (Rickham and Mawdsley 1966). 203 infants born with spina bifida aperta lesions in Liverpool between 1960 and 1962 (an incidence of 3.7 per 1,000 total births) were studied; 46 were recorded as stillborn (23 per cent) and 27 (13 per cent) died within 24 hours of birth and were assumed to be untreatable. Of the remaining 130, 100 were referred and operated upon, and the 30 unoperated cases all died except two. 71 of the 100 operated patients survived three years or more, and, after the exclusion of the meningoceles and myelomeningoceles which were already covered with reasonable skin at birth, there were 64 long-term survivors (49 per cent) for later assessment. This figure has been compared with a deduced 15.8 per cent of the first-day survivors with both open and skin-covered myelomeningoceles from the South Wales series.

63 of the 64 survivors from the Liverpool series were later analysed for the quality

of their survival (Mawdsley *et al.* 1967) at a time when the youngest was five years of age. 17 of these children were mentally and physically normal, nine had only minor handicaps. 30 children had major handicaps (physical, physico-mental or mental only) and seven were considered to be vegetative (four of these were children with large encephaloceles and microcephalus, and not true spina bifida aperta lesions).

In Cambridge, the policy of early assessment and surgical treatment of infants born with spina bifida aperta lesions was adopted from July 1963 onwards. The 96 infants seen between that date and June 1967 were personally examined at various intervals and the results of their treatment assessed (Brocklehurst 1968*b*). It was found, by obtaining the Registrar General's figures for notifications of spina bifida (live and stillborn) in 1964 and 1965 for the East Anglian region, and by a field survey throughout that region, that the rate was 1.16 and 1.60 per 1,000 births for those two years: throughout the period studied the average number of 26 a year seen at Cambridge represented the majority of the infants born per annum in the region after the deduction of a 25 per cent stillbirth rate, and five per annum who were considered too disabled to be referred. 84 of these infants were operated upon, 79 of these within the first 48 hours of birth, and at the time of the assessment 69 patients were still alive. Life table calculations made from the numbers of infants actually referred for assessment and treatment showed a 65 per cent chance of survival up to two years, and a 56 per cent chance up to four years. These figures, which do not include encephaloceles but do include meningoceles, may be compared with the Liverpool and South Wales experience.

The quality of survival of 113 patients operated upon at Cambridge within 48 hours of birth between July 1963 and January 1971 was assessed between March 1971 and March 1972, when the children were aged between fifteen months and seven years and eight months. There were 80 survivors (71 per cent), and of the 33 deaths, 23 had occurred in the first year (20 per cent). The over-all disability of the survivors was minimal in six per cent, moderate in 40 per cent, severe in 39 per cent, and very severe in 15 per cent (Hunt *et al.* 1973). A good correlation was found between the sensory level as determined by the general response of the infant to pinprick (see Chapter 6) and the degree of ultimate disability. A high sensory level (T10 and above) and an intermediate sensory level (T11 to L3) correlated with the moderate-severe and very severe disabilities, as did also an open myeloschisis, a head size greater than the 90th percentile at birth, a lesion anatomically in the thoraco-lumbar region, and paralysed quadriceps muscles.

In Sheffield, a large number of infants with spina bifida lesions have been assessed and treated, the majority within 48 hours of birth. An initial detailed assessment of results of 526 patients with open spina bifida aperta lesions (myelomeningoceles or myeloschisis) was made (Sharrard *et al.* 1967). Unfortunately they were divided into six groups according to the time at which they were seen and the time at which they were operated upon or not. This produces some difficulties in the analysis and comparability with other series, but it is clear that the cumulative survival of the groups seen and operated upon in the first four days of life is considerably higher at 36 months (51.2 per cent) than in those seen later and treated by delayed closure or no closure (32.2 per cent).

169

Effect of Early Closure upon Lower Limb Movement

This aspect of the quality of the survivors after early closure of spina bifida aperta lesions was very critically considered after the publication by Sharrard *et al.* (1963) of the improvement in lower limb muscle function following the procedure. In the initial communication, specified groups of muscles were considered and scored by grading them according to the M.R.C. (Medical Research Council) system of 0 to 5. Later, the pre- and post-operative numerical scores were added together and a comparison made between the early-closure series and no-closure series. There were serious limitations to this method of assessment, since the muscles were being considered only in relation to their lower motor neurone control and the absence or presence of lower motor neurone lesions. As scores could only be obtained by direct handling of the muscles and stimulation of the overlying skin and adjacent joints, some inaccuracy in the numerical scores seemed inevitable. In the 1967 assessment (Sharrard *et al. opus cit.*) a more functional grading was used, based upon the assessment of power in the various muscle groups: grade 0 indicated complete paralysis, and grade 5 normal lower limbs; grades 2 and 3 indicated paralysis with the possibility of walking aided by reconstructive operations and support. These assessments were still directly related to the functions of muscle groups under lower motor neurone control, without the determination of spastic paralysis of the upper motor neurone lesion type. By this means of assessment, the patients who underwent early closure showed a preservation of the functional grades of paralysis, so that in the survivors assessed at three years, 24 per cent had grades 0 to 1, 42 per cent grades 2 to 3 and 34 per cent grades 4 and 5. The no-closure group consisted of 60 per cent, 28 per cent and 12 per cent respectively in these grades.

Neurological assessment of lower limb movement in infants with spina bifida that recognises upper and lower motor neurone lesions, and some of the varieties and mixtures outlined in Chapters 4 and 6, has been applied to the neonatal infant before and after operative closure within the first 24 hours of life. In a study of 25 infants, Brocklehurst *et al.* (1967*a, b*) showed that the majority, when assessed three months after their operation, had similar or less lower limb movement under upper motor neurone control than they had shown pre-operatively, with the exception of five patients who appeared to show significant improvement. The later assessment of these patients, however, showed a return to the pre-operative level or below in all excepting one; early closure appeared to have prevented the death of the infants and to have preserved the useful leg movements with which they were born, but not to have led to any significant recovery.

Duckworth and Brown (1970) studied the patients at Sheffield in further detail. They first of all demonstrated that their clinical assessment of muscle activity, *i.e.* an inspection during which the child was kept alert by gentle stimulation such as stroking the skin or gently moving the limbs (there is no mention of whether or not this movement was being studied at levels below the general sensory level, and in segments which might be subjected to upper motor neurone lesions) could be related to muscle activity as detected by electromyography with a 70 per cent to 80 per cent agreement. They then studied 16 children and found that in three of them virtually normal lower limb activity was present and was maintained for up to six months, that in another three there was no pre-operative spontaneous muscle function (some muscle groups were shown to respond to faradic stimulation), and that at one year muscle activity was the same as at birth, and spontaneous activity never developed in the muscles which did not show response to faradism at birth. In a third group of nine patients there was little or no spontaneous activity at birth, there was a faradic response in nearly all of the muscle groups, and after closure there appeared to be gradual improvement in muscle function—up to two to three months when judged clinically. Thereafter, the spontaneous activity declined, and by 12 months the over-all picture was almost exactly the same as at birth. This study from Sheffield shows clearly that muscle function under lower motor neurone control will appear and improve after closure of the plaque, but will later undergo deterioration, and this is in keeping with the neuropathology of these lesions as described in Chapters 3 and 4. In the myeloschisis or myelodysplasia lesions of the spinal cord, there is ample lower motor neurone innervation of muscle groups which lie caudal to the general sensory level of the spinal lesion, and many of these groups will show spontaneous and reflex activity at birth. This lower motor neurone activity can be so striking that it appears to be as vigorous as the voluntary movements of the child's upper limbs, and it is sometimes difficult to distinguish these. Such activity disappears easily if the child is cold or if the plaque degenerates, and is enhanced by early closure of the plaque. Direct muscle power assessment, faradic stimulation and, to some extent, electro-myography will detect this lower motor neurone activity, and only careful clinical assessment with attention to the general sensory level, combined with electro-myography in certain difficult cases will elucidate the upper motor neurone lesion. These later studies which confirm that the effect of early closure is to preserve the useful leg movements with which the infants are born in no way refutes the equally certain observations that exposure, drying and infection of the open spina bifida lesion will lead to true neurological deterioration in addition to the more obvious loss of lower motor neurone function.

The quality of survival of the spina bifida patients treated at Sheffield has been most fully analysed by Lorber (1971). Only one per cent of the initial admissions and four per cent of the total survivors have no handicap; 15 per cent have a moderate total handicap; 49 per cent are severely handicapped; and a further 33 per cent are extremely impaired. Nearly 40 per cent of the handicapped survivors were able to be schooled in an ordinary school, and the remainder required special care.

Summary of Results of Early Operation on All Patients
Accurate comparison of figures obtained from differently constituted series is difficult, but a generalised summary of the results of indiscriminate early closure can now be put forward.

The initial mortality can be expected to remain as low as one per cent in centres where early closure is the customary procedure; survival of the post-operative period with the problems of acute hydrocephalus and its treatment is about 85 per cent, and 80 per cent should reach three months. Survival up to one year is between 60 per cent and 70 per cent and to three years about 60 per cent; the five-year survival rate from early closure of all patients presenting within the first 48 hours of birth is about 50 per cent. The figures that are available for later follow-up, *i.e.* to seven years, show a survival rate of about 40 per cent.

Taking L1 as the borderline level, 40 to 50 per cent will have high lesions, and taking L3 as the level this rises to between 50 and 60 per cent. Following early closure, the neurological function of the lower limbs is preserved, and at the three-year stage at least 25 per cent are totally paralysed, and a further 25 per cent nearly so. Of the remainder, under 25 per cent are without significant lower limb dysfunction, which leaves a core of about 25 per cent requiring very active orthopaedic care to achieve walking.

Ninety per cent of the infants presenting initially will have neurologically abnormal bladders, and for the first year of life many will be beset by recurrent urinary tract infections. A few will develop hydronephrosis and pyelonephrosis during this time. At the late follow-up, 17 per cent have normal continence, 56 per cent are incontinent, and 27 per cent have ileal loops. The upper urinary tract has been preserved as normal in 57 per cent of the survivors, but the remainder have sustained permanent damage from chronic pyelonephritis and hydronephrosis. Hydrocephalus is likely to occur in 90 per cent of the patients, and 75 to 80 per cent will require treatment by shunting procedure. The average revision rate for these shunts is between 30 and 50 per cent in the first year, 50 to 75 per cent in the second year, and almost all will have been revised at least once by the fourth year. The survival of patients who have not actually required a shunting procedure for hydrocephalus is 89 per cent at seven years and the I.Q. range 50 to 129 (average 87). Survival of patients with hydrocephalus which has required shunting is 37 per cent and the I.Q. range 10 to 125 (average 79) (Lorber 1971).

Results of Early Operation on Selected Cases

In Edinburgh, a selective policy in the treatment of spina bifida infants has been pursued since 1965 and the results in 163 of these patients have been reported (Stark and Drummond 1972). 95 per cent of the infants were seen within 12 hours of birth, and were neurologically assessed in a manner similar to that outlined in Chapter 6. Using criteria based upon the height of the neurological lesion, skull enlargement present at birth, and associated severe spinal deformities, only 47.8 per cent were operated on. With few exceptions, the unoperated infants died in the first three months of life, and more than 70 per cent of the treated infants were alive at six years. The incidence of severe physical disability, upper urinary tract damage and severe mental handicap were each more than 20 per cent lower than that found in the later analysis of the Sheffield series of unselected early closures.

From 1971, a policy of early selection of patients for surgical treatment was commenced at Sheffield, and the initial results of this have been recently published (Lorber 1973a). Of 37 newborn infants referred within 24 hours of birth, 25 were rejected for surgical treatment because of the gross paralysis, the thoraco-lumbar site of the lesion, congenital kyphosis, an enlarged head at birth, or a cerebral birth injury or multiple congenital defects. Death occurred in all of these infants within nine months of age. Of the 12 treated infants, 10 were surviving at the time of review; three of these were fully normal, seven had slight paraplegia, and three were incontinent with moderate paraplegia. Four of the surviving infants had no hydrocephalus.

A selective policy was adopted in Carshalton in 1971. Infants with a kyphosis, very high lesions, scoliosis, abnormal ribs and other congenital abnormalities were not operated upon, and infants with a total lower limb paralysis or gross hydrocephalus at birth had the back lesion closed but no resuscitative treatment was undertaken if a crisis occurred. The remaining infants were treated fully. The percentage of patients surviving one year fell from 85 per cent in 1970 to 67.5 per cent in 1971, and 50 per cent in 1972, the striking change occurring half way through 1971 when the selective policy was adopted. The quality of the survivors was improved (Colliss 1972).

Putting these results together again, it seems that of 100 children born with spina bifida aperta lesions with neurological involvement and who survive the first 24 hours, somewhat more than 50 per cent will be paralysed from the knees downwards, and if no active surgical treatment is undertaken the five-year survival is around 16 per cent and half of these have moderate or severe disabilities. Unselected early surgical treatment puts the survival rate up to around 40 per cent, but about three-quarters of these children are severely handicapped. Early selection for surgical treatment, based upon well-established criteria, will result in between 50 and 60 per cent of the patients being rejected (nearly all of whom will die in the first year). The survival rate of the remaining 40 per cent is likely to be high, and could be estimated at perhaps between 60 and 75 per cent by five years in centres specialising in the care of these infants. One third of these will have some mild to moderate impairment, and the remainder will be minimally impaired or normal.

A Selection of Type of Treatment Based on Prognosis

The experience of the last 10 years has provided an ample background of knowledge of the nature of spina bifida and the results of surgical treatment. Preservation of life is possible in the majority of infants with the spina bifida aperta lesions if active treatment is undertaken within a few hours of birth, but those who survive into later childhood include many with a handicap such as mental retardation, severe physical immobility or a combination of these, with incontinence, renal failure and severe spinal deformities. This situation can be altered only by witholding surgical treatment from those infants with a known poor prognosis.

In the clinical assessment of the newborn infant with a spina bifida aperta lesion outlined in Chapter 6, the infants were categorised in relationship to the site and severity of the spinal lesion, the various types of accompanying neurological deficit and other associated conditions. The decision to undertake surgical treatment should be based upon the likelihood that the infant will have reasonably normal mental function if any subsequent hydrocephalus is adequately treated, will have some function of the lower limbs so that ambulation might be achieved, and the infant should not have severe accompanying congenital malformations such as congenital kyphus or scoliosis, congenital heart lesions or severe gastro-intestinal deformities. Expressed in another way, the newborn infant with an open spina bifida lesion should not be operated upon if:

173

(1) there is no lower limb movement under normal upper motor neurone control (*i.e.* there is a paraplegia from L1 downwards);

(2) there is clinically established hydrocephalus at birth (enlarged skull circumference);

(3) there is an associated lumbar kyphosis or severe scoliosis;

(4) there are serious congenital malformations in other systems;

(5) the general neurological state of the infant is poor (from birth trauma or anoxia).

Infants and children presenting with spina bifida occulta lesions (see Chapter 7) should always be considered for surgical treatment; those with a congenital dermal sinus with the attendant risk of infection, and those with cord or conus compression should be treated urgently, and the other patients considered for prophylactic treatment.

The Difficult Decisions

Decisions should be made individually for each patient and should not be just the result of gross categorisations. The accurate clinical, neurological and radiological assessment of the infant in a centre that has experience with these problems is the first requirement, and the nature of the condition and the particular prognosis should be explained simply to one or both parents. In the case of an infant with a limited spina bifida aperta lesion and a relatively good prognosis, surgical treatment should be strongly recommended to the parents or guardian, while at the same time the likely problems of the future such as hydrocephalus, lower limb paresis, incontinence, and their treatment should be discussed. It is unusual for a parent to be able to assimilate much of this at such an early stage, but since a rapid decision has to be made if the infant's neurological state is to be preserved, many parents will be content to accept the advice of the surgeon or paediatrician regarding treatment. It is important to let the parents know the infant's limitations and likely disability prior to the operation, and to explain that the operation cannot restore neurological function which has never developed.

The infant with a severe lesion and a poor prognosis on the criteria mentioned above should be considered in like detail with the parents and nursing staff, and the nature of the present and likely future situation explained. Surgical treatment should not be advocated, and the management of the infant should be undertaken along medical lines as described in Chapter 6. Responsibility and communication between parents, nurses and medical staff should continue, and the infant should remain in hospital until death occurs, unless parents specifically request to take it home for brief periods of care.

In some circumstances a parent or doctor may feel that life should be preserved at all costs and insist upon surgical treatment being undertaken—at least as far as closure of the back wound. This should be resisted, because although it may make the nursing treatment apparently easier, it postpones the ultimate death of such a severely impaired infant and increases the length of suffering endured both by the infant and the parents.

Some parents, particularly those with a large family or other problem children, or difficult home circumstances, may find the prospect of a child with even moderate limitations forbidding, and may firmly refuse the treatment. In these circumstances the infant should receive the same medical treatment as those which have been more formally rejected for operation. The occasional parent or guardian who is sufficiently appalled at a minor disability or defect to refuse treatment of a child with a relatively good prognosis should be firmly persuaded that responsibility is primarily to the infant and, in this respect, that treatment should be undertaken which is in the best interest of its future.

It is not uncommon when faced with a robust infant with only one of the contra-indications to surgical treatment described above, e.g. total paraplegia but no hydrocephalus, or spina bifida aperta and a treatable additional congenital anomaly, for both parents and surgeon to incline towards a decision in favour of surgical treatment and the preservation of life on the grounds that in this individual situation more happiness would ensue than the alternative of leaving the parents with the lingering regret that not enough was done for their child.

These decisions are sometimes difficult and are the subject of much individual variation in ethical concepts and comprehension; the team of the parents, nursing staff, paediatrician and surgeon should co-operate fully in whatever final decision is reached and in the subsequent medical or surgical management (see Chapter 12).

CHAPTER 14

Counting the Cost

The renewed interest in spina bifida and the widespread efforts to treat the condition during the last 10 years have led to a more accurate appreciation of the wide spectrum of pathology which accompanies it and of the necessity for a comprehensive inter-disciplinary approach to its management. The cost of such treatment, in the widest implications of the word, is now becoming clear. The results of modern comprehensive treatment have been outlined in Chapter 13 and show that a considerable percentage of the present-day survivors are extremely limited, both physically and mentally, and the effect of this upon patient and parents has been discussed in Chapter 12. The personal experience of many who have worked with children with these conditions and of many parents who have cared for them at home is that few would have wished to embark upon the initial treatment in many cases had they known the ultimate severity of the limitations and the load which such prolonged treatment imposes upon both child and parents.

Financial Cost

To the cost in terms of mental and physical suffering must be added that of the financial expense borne by parents, insurance companies, or some such third party as the community at large via the health and welfare services. Calculations based upon relatively recent experience in England show the average cost per initial hospitalisation to be £400; similar calculations for the U.S.A. give a range of $244 to $6,539 (£100 to £2,500), with an average of $2,305 (just under £1,000). The average cost for a series of readmissions studied in the U.S.A. was just over $2,484 (just greater than £1,000), with a range of $75 to $8,638 (Brocklehurst and Barnett 1972). It has also been estimated that each child will incur further prolonged expense if kept in an institution, but this is obviously reduced when full comprehensive treatment of the child has resulted in a degree of disability compatible with management at home in between the recurrent hospital admissions. The pursuit of a policy of unselected early surgical treatment (see Chapter 13) creates a heavy economic burden which was calculated to be something like 3.3 million pounds per year for England (Lightowler 1971).

The Worthwhile Child

The preservation into later childhood of that group of children with good or reasonable mental function and legs upon which they can walk or ambulate in some fashion is undoubtedly a worthwhile undertaking. Such children are not only rewarding to their parents but are capable of education and a gainful occupation in later life. It should be the aim of every clinician concerned with the management of infants and children with spina bifida lesions to see that accurate assessment and full detailed and comprehensive management is available from the time of birth onwards, so that the maximal achievements of these patients can be realised, and, at the same time, to be prepared to accept that in many cases the maldevelopment is of such a degree that it imposes an unacceptable burden upon the infant, parents and society. The recognition of this degree of severity in any particular infant, and the decision not to undertake certain courses of medical treatment which would preserve life, is a responsibility in the use of present-day knowledge and skills which both patient and society deserves.

REFERENCES

Ahlfeld, J. F. (1880) *Die Missbildungen des Menschen. Eine systematische Darstellung der beim Menschen angeboren vorkommenden Missbildungen und Erklärung ihrer Entstehungsweise.* Leipzig: F. W. Grunow, p. 294.

Allan, L. D., Ferguson-Smith, H. A., Donald, I., Sweet, E. M., Gibson, A. A. M. (1973) 'Amniotic-fluid alpha-fetoprotein in the antenatal diagnosis of spina bifida.' *Lancet,* **ii,** 522.

Alliaume, A. (1950) 'Fractures des os longs dans les myéloméningocèles.' *Archives Françaises de Pédiatrie,* **7,** 294.

Alter, M. (1962) 'Anencephalus, hydrocephalus and spina bifida. Epidemiology, with special reference to a survey in Charleston, S.C.' *Archives of Neurology,* **7,** 411.

Alvord, E. C. (1961) 'The pathology of hydrocephalus.' *In* Fields, W. S., Desmond, M. M. (Eds.) *Disorders of the Developing Nervous system.* Springfield, Ill.: C. C. Thomas.

Ardran, G. M., Cope, V., Essenhigh, D. M., Tuckey, M. (1967) 'Observations on the function of the bladder neck and urethra in dogs.' *British Journal of Urology,* **39,** 334.

Arey, L. B. (1954) *Developmental Anatomy. A Textbook and Laboratory Manual of Embryology,* 6th ed. Philadelphia: W. B. Saunders.

Arnold, J. (1894) 'Myelocyste, Transposition von Gewebskeimen und Sympodie.' *Beiträge zur pathologischen Anatomie und zur allgemeinen Pathologie,* **16,** 1.

Badell-Ribera, A., Shulman, K., Paddock, N. (1966) 'The relationship of non-progressive hydrocephalus to intellectual functioning in children with spina bifida cystica.' *Pediatrics,* **37,** 787.

Bailey, R. R., Gower, P. E., Roberts, A. P., de Wardener, H. E. (1971) 'Prevention of urinary tract infection with low-dose nitrofurantoin.' *Lancet,* **ii,** 1112.

Baker, R. H., Sharrard, W. J. W. (1973) 'Correction of lordoscoliosis in spina bifida by multiple spinal osteotomy and fusion with Dwyer fixation: a preliminary report.' *Developmental Medicine and Child Neurology,* suppl. 29, 12.

Barratt, T. M. (1974) *In* Alken, C. E., Dix, V. W., Weyrauch, H. M., Wildbolz, E. (Eds.) *Encyclopaedia of Urology,* vol. XV (Suppl.) *Urology in Childhood.* Berlin: Springer.

Barry, A., Patten, B. M., Stewart, B. H. (1957) 'Possible factors in the development of the Arnold-Chiari malformation.' *Journal of Neurosurgery,* **14,** 285.

Barson, A. J. (1965) 'Radiological studies of spina bifida cystica. The phenomenon of congenital lumbar kyphosis.' *British Journal of Radiology,* **38,** 294.

—— (1970a) 'Spina bifida; the significance of the level and extent of the defect to the morphogenesis.' *Developmental Medicine and Child Neurology,* **12,** 129.

—— (1970b) 'The vertebral level of termination of the spinal cord during normal and abnormal development.' *Journal of Anatomy,* **106,** 489.

Bartelmez, G. W., Dekaban, A. S. (1962) 'The early development of the human brain.' *Contributions to Embryology,* **37,** 13.

Bates, C. P., Corney, C. E. (1971) 'Synchronous cine/pressure/flow cystography: a method of routine urodynamic investigation.' *British Journal of Radiology,* **44,** 44.

Bendix, S. (1973) 'The administrative and social management of the family with a newborn spina bifida infant.' Presented to the 17th Annual Meeting of the Society for Research into Hydrocephalus and Spina Bifida.

Bering, E. A. (1962) 'Circulation of the cerebrospinal fluid. Demonstration of the choroid plexuses as the generator of the force for flow of fluid and ventricular enlargement.' *Journal of Neurosurgery,* **19,** 405.

Blaauw, G. (1970) 'The dural sinuses and the veins in the midline of the brain in myelomeningocele.' *Developmental Medicine and Child Neurology,* suppl. 22, 12.

Blazé, J. B., Forrest, D. M., Tsingoglou, S. (1971) 'Atriotomy using the Holter shunt in hydrocephalus.' *Developmental Medicine and Child Neurology,* suppl. 25, 27.

Blockey, N. J. (1971) 'Aids for crippled children.' *Developmental Medicine and Child Neurology,* **13,** 216.

Bogash, M., Kohler, F. P., Scott, R. H., Murphy, J. J. (1959) 'Replacement of the urinary bladder by a plastic reservoir with mechanical valves.' *Surgical Forum,* **10,** 900.

Boyce, W. H., Lathem, J. E., Hunt, L. D. (1964) 'Research related to the development of an artificial electrical stimulator for the paralyzed human bladder: a review.' *Journal of Urology,* **91,** 41.

Bradley, W. E., Timm, G. W., Chou, S. N. (1971) 'A decade of experience with electronic stimulation of the micturition reflex.' *Urologia Internationalis,* **26,** 283.

Bricker, E. M. (1950) 'Bladder substitution after pelvic evisceration.' *Surgical Clinics of North America,* **30,** 1511.

—— Sutcliffe, R. G. (1972) 'Alpha fetoprotein in the antenatal diagnosis of anencephaly and spina bifida.' *Lancet,* **ii,** 197.

178

Brock, D. J. H., Bolton, A. E., Scrimgeour, J. B. (1974) 'Prenatal diagnosis of spina bifida and anencephaly through maternal plasma—alpha-fetoprotein measurement.' *Lancet,* **i,** 767.

Brocklehurst, G. (1968*a*) 'The significance of the pathogenesis of spina bifida to its treatment.' M. Chir. Thesis. University of Cambridge.

—— (1968*b*) 'Use of radio-iodinated serum albumin in the study of cerebrospinal fluid flow.' *Journal of Neurology, Neurosurgery and Psychiatry,* **31,** 162.

—— (1969*a*) 'A quantitative study of a spina bifida foetus.' *Journal of Pathology and Bacteriology,* **99,** 205.

—— (1969*b*) 'The development of the human cerebrospinal fluid pathway with particular reference to the roof of the fourth ventricle.' *Journal of Anatomy,* **105,** 467.

—— (1971) 'The pathogenesis of spina bifida: a study of the relationship between observation, hypothesis and surgical incentive.' *Developmental Medicine and Child Neurology,* **13,** 147.

—— (1972) 'Further observations on the use of radio-iodinated serum albumin in the study of CSF flow.' *In* Harbert, J. C., McCullough, D. C., Luessenhop, A. J., Di Chiro, G. (Eds.) *Cisternography and Hydrocephalus: a Symposium.* Springfield, Ill.: C. C. Thomas.

—— (1974*a*) 'Transcallosal third ventriculo-chiasmatic cisternography—a new approach to hydrocephalus.' *Surgical Neurology,* **2,** 109.

—— (1974*b*) The Foramen of Magendie. Carins Essay.

—— Barnett, B., (1972) 'The comprehensive care of patients with spina bifida.' *Journal of the Kentucky Medical Association,* **70,** 860.

—— Gleave, J. R. W., Lewin, W. S. (1967*a*) 'Early closure of myelomeningocele with special reference to leg movement.' *British Medical Journal,* **i,** 666.

—— —— —— (1967*b*) 'Early closure of myelomeningocele with special reference to leg movement.' *Developmental Medicine and Child Neurology,* suppl. 13, 51.

—— —— Millar, R. A., Adams, A. K. (1967*c*) 'Hydrocephalus: electrocardiographic localisation of the catheter in ventriculo-atrial shunts.' *Archives of Disease in Childhood,* **42,** 166.

Brown, M., Wickham, J. E. A. (1969) 'The urethral pressure profile.' *British Journal of Urology,* **41,** 211.

Buisson, J. S., Hamblen, D. L. (1972) 'Electromyographic assessment of the transplanted ilio-psoas muscle in spina bifida cystica.' *Developmental Medicine and Child Neurology,* suppl. 27, 29.

Caldwell, K. P. S. (1963) 'The electrical control of sphincter incompetence.' *Lancet,* **ii,** 174.

—— Flack, F. C., Broad, A. F. (1965) 'Urinary incontinence following spinal cord injury treated by electronic implant.' *Lancet,* **i,** 846.

Cameron, A. H. (1957) 'The Arnold-Chiari and other neuroanatomical malformations associated with spina bifida.' *Journal of Pathology and Bacteriology,* **73,** 195.

Carlsson, C. A., Sundin, T. (1967) 'Reconstruction of efferent pathways to the urinary bladder in a paraplegic child.' *Review of Surgery,* **24,** 73.

Carroll, M. C., Sharrard, W. J. W. (1972) 'Long-term follow-up of posterior iliopsoas transplantation for paralytic dislocation of the hip.' *Journal of Bone and Joint Surgery,* **54A,** 551.

Carter, C. O. (1974) 'Clues to the aetiology of neural tube malformations.' *Developmental Medicine and Child Neurology,* suppl. 32, 3.

—— Roberts, J. A. F. (1967) 'The risk of recurrence after two children with central-nervous-system malformations.' *Lancet,* **i,** 306.

Chantraine, A., Stevenaert, A., Timmermans, L. (1967) 'Electromyographic study before and after operation in spina bifida with myelomeningocele: a preliminary report.' *Developmental Medicine and Child Neurology,* suppl. 13, 136.

Chiari, H. (1891) 'Über Veränderungen des Kleinhirns infolge von Hydrocephalie des Grosshirns.' *Deutsche medizinische Wochenschrift,* **17,** 1172.

—— (1896) 'Über die Veränderungen des Kleinhirns, des Pons und der Medulla Oblongata infolge von congenitaler Hydrocephalie des Grosshirns.' *Denkschriften der Akademie der Wissenschaften, Wien,* **63,** 71.

Cholmeley, J. A. (1953) 'Elmslie's operation for the calcaneus foot.' *Journal of Bone and Joint Surgery,* **35B,** 46.

Cleland, J. (1883) 'Contribution to the study of spina bifida, encephalocele and anencephalus.' *Journal of Anatomy and Physiology,* **17,** 257.

Cohen, H., Davies, S. (1937) 'The development of the cerebrospinal spaces and choroid plexuses in the chick.' *Journal of Anatomy,* **72,** 23.

—— —— (1938) 'The morphology and permeability of the roof of the fourth ventricle in some mammalian embryos.' *Journal of Anatomy,* **72,** 430.

Colliss, V. R. (1972) 'The effects of selective treatment of myelomeningocele on a neonatal unit.' *Developmental Medicine and Child Neurology,* suppl. 27, 34.

179

Comar, A. E. (1967) *In* Boyarsky, S. (Ed.) *The Neurogenic Bladder.* Baltimore: Williams and Wilkins, p. 191.

Cook, R. C. M., Lister, J., Zachary, R. B. (1968) 'Operative management of the neurogenic bladder in children—diversion through intestinal conduits.' *Surgery,* **63,** 825.

Cooper, D. G. W. (1968) 'Bladder studies in children with neurogenic incontinence, with comments on the place of pelvic floor stimulation.' *British Journal of Urology,* **40,** 157.

Cotugno, D. (1764) *De Ischiade Nervosa Commentarius.* Naples: Frat. Simonii.

Craig, W. A., Kunin, C. M., Degroot, J. (1973) 'Evaluation of new urinary tract infection screening devices.' *Applied Microbiology,* **26,** 196.

Cruess, R. L., Turner, N. S. (1970) 'Paralysis of hip abductor muscles in spina bifida. Results of treatment by the Mustard procedure.' *Journal of Bone and Joint Surgery,* **52A,** 1364.

Cudmore, R. E., Zachary, R. B. (1970) 'The renogram and the renal tract in spina bifida.' *Developmental Medicine and Child Neurology,* suppl. 22, 24.

Curtis, B. H., Fisher, R. L. (1969) 'Congenital hyperextension with anterior subluxation of the knee. Surgical treatment and long-term observations.' *Journal of Bone and Joint Surgery,* **51A,** 255.

Cushing, H. (1926) *Studies in Intracranial Physiology and Surgery. The Third Circulation; the Hypophysis; the Gliomas.* London: Oxford University Press.

Damanski, M. (1967) 'The paraplegic bladder.' *Hospital Medicine,* **2,** 39.

Dandy, W. E. (1918) 'Extirpation of the choroid plexus of the lateral ventricles in communicating hydrocephalus.' *American Surgeon,* **68,** 569.

—— (1919) 'Experimental hydrocephalus.' *American Surgeon,* **70,** 129.

—— (1922) 'An operative procedure for hydrocephalus.' *Johns Hopkins Hospital Bulletin,* **33,** 189.

—— Blackfan, K. D. (1913) 'An experimental and clinical study of internal hydrocephalus.' *Journal of the American Medical Association,* **61,** 2216.

—— —— (1914) 'Internal hydrocephalus. An experimental, clinical and pathological study.' *American Journal of the Diseases of Children,* **8,** 406.

—— —— (1917) 'Internal hydrocephalus.' *American Journal of the Diseases of Children,* **14,** 424.

Daniel, P. M., Strich, S. J. (1958) 'Some observations on the congenital deformity of the central nervous system known as the Arnold-Chiari malformation.' *Journal of Neuropathology and Experimental Neurology,* **17,** 255.

D'Arcy, E. (1968) 'Congenital defects: mothers' first reactions to information.' *British Medical Journal,* **iii,** 796.

de Lange, S. A. (1974) 'Selection for treatment of patients with spina bifida aperta.' *Developmental Medicine and Child Neurology,* suppl. 32, 27.

Doran, P. A., Guthkelch, a. N. (1961) 'Studies in spina bifida cystica. I. General survey and reassessment of the problem.' *Journal of Neurology, Neurosurgery and Psychiatry,* **24,** 331.

Dorner, S. (1973) 'Psychological and social problems of families of adolescent spina bifida patients: a preliminary report.' *Developmental Medicine and Child Neurology,* suppl. 29, 24.

—— (1974) 'Some problems of families with an adolescent spina bifida patient.' *Developmental Medicine and Child Neurology,* suppl. 32, 153 (Summary).

Drennan, J. C. (1970) The role of muscles in the development of human lumbar kyphosis. *Developmental Medicine and Child Neurology,* suppl. 22, 33.

—— Sharrard, W. J. W. (1971) 'The pathological anatomy of convex pes valgus.' *Journal of Bone and Joint Surgery,* **53B,** 455.

Duckworth, T., Brown, B. H. (1970) 'Changes in muscle activity following early closure of myelomeningocele.' *Developmental Medicine and Child Neurology,* suppl. 22, 39.

—— Smith, T. W. D. (1974) 'The treatment of paralytic convex pes valgus.' *Journal of Bone and Joint Surgery,* **56B,** 305.

—— Sharrard, W. J. W., Lister, J., Seymour, N. (1968) 'Hemimyelocele.' *Developmental Medicine and Child Neurology,* suppl.16, 69.

Duthie, E. J. W., Stark, G. D. (1974) 'Catheters for continence: a preliminary report on their trial in myelomeningocele.' *Developmental Medicine and Child Neurology,* suppl. 32, 31.

Dwyer, A. F., Newton, N. C., Sherwood, A. A. (1969) 'An anterior approach to scoliosis. A preliminary report.' *Clinical Orthopaedics,* **62,** 192.

Dwyer, F. C. (1959) 'Osteotomy of the calcaneum for pes cavus.' *Journal of Bone and Joint Surgery,* **41B,** 80.

Eckstein, H. B. (1968) 'The neurogenic bladder and urinary diversion.' *In* Williams, D. I. (Ed.), *Paediatric Urology.* London: Butterworths.

—— (1974) *In* Williams, D. I. (Ed.), *Urology in Childhood. Encyclopaedia of Urology,* vol. XV. suppl. Berlin: Springer.

—— Cooper, D. G. W., Howard, E. R., Pike, J. (1967) 'Cause of death in children with meningomyelocele or hydrocephalus.' *Archives of Disease in Childhood,* **42,** 163.

—— Kapila, L. (1970) 'Cutaneous ureterostomy.' *British Journal of Urology,* **42,** 306.

Edwards, L., Malvern, J. (1972a) 'Electronic control of incontinence: a critical review of the present situation.' *British Journal of Urology,* **44,** 467.

—— —— (1972b) 'The urethral pressure profile: theoretical considerations and clinical application.' *British Journal of Urology,* **46,** 325.

Ellis, F., Parker, J., Hills, M. (1964) 'Experimental electrical stimulation of the bladder.' *British Journal of Surgery,* **51,** 857.

Ellis, H. L. (1974) 'Parental involvement in the decision to treat spina bifida cystica.' *British Medical Journal,* **i,** 369.

Emery, J. L. (1974) 'Deformity of the aqueduct of Sylvius in children with hydrocephalus and myelomeningocele.' *Developmental Medicine and Child Neurology,* suppl. 32, 40.

—— Lendon, R. G. (1969) 'Lipomas of the cauda equina and other fatty tumours related to neurospinal dysraphism.' *Developmental Medicine and Child Neurology,* suppl. 20, 62.

—— —— (1972) 'Clinical implications of cord lesions in neurospinal dysraphism.' *Developmental Medicine and Child Neurology,* suppl. 27, 45.

—— Levick, R. K. (1966) 'The movement of the brain stem and vessels around the brain stem in children with hydrocephalus and the Arnold-Chiari deformity.' *Developmental Medicine and Child Neurology,* suppl. 11, 49.

—— Naik, D. R. (1968) 'Spinal cord segment lengths in children with meningomyelocele and the "Cleland-Arnold-Chiari" deformity.' *British Journal of Radiology,* **41,** 287.

—— Svitok, I. (1968) 'Inter-hemispherical distances in congenital hydrocephalus associated with meningomyelocele.' *Developmental Medicine and Child Neurology,* suppl. 15, 21.

Engel, R. M. E., Schirmer, H. K. A. (1974) 'Pudendal neurectomy in neurogenic bladder.' *Journal of Urology,* **112,** 57.

Erdohazi, M., Eckstein, H. B., Crome, L. (1966) 'Pulmonary embolisation as a complication of ventriculo-atrial shunts inserted for hydrocephalus.' *Developmental Medicine and Child Neurology,* suppl. 11, 36.

Evans, D. (1961) 'Relapsed club foot.' *Journal of Bone and Joint Surgery,* **43B,** 722.

Eyring, E. J., Wanken, J. J., Sayers, M. P. (1972) 'Spine osteotomy for kyphosis in myelomeningocele.' *Clinical Orthopaedics,* **88,** 24.

Fairley, K. F., Bond, A. G., Brown, R. B., Habersberger, P. (1967) 'Simple test to determine the site of urinary tract infection.' *Lancet,* **ii,** 427.

Fernandez-Serrats, A. A., Guthkelch, A. N., Parker, S. A. (1967) 'The prognosis of open myelocele with a note on a trial of Laurence's operation.' *Developmental Medicine and Child Neurology,* suppl. 13, 65.

Field, B. (1972) 'The child with spina bifida: medical and social aspects of the problems of the child with multiple handicaps and his family.' *Medical Journal of Australia,* **2,** 1284.

Fleming, C. P. (1967) 'The verbal behaviour of hydrocephalic children.' *Developmental Medicine and Child Neurology,* suppl. 15, 74.

Forbes, M., Underwood, J., Emery, J. L. (1969) 'The intrinsic innervation of the dilated ureter in children with myelomeningocele.' *Developmental Medicine and Child Neurology,* suppl. 20, 49.

Forrest, D. M. (1974) 'The use of the Foley catheter for long-term urine collection in girls.' *Developmental Medicine and Child Neurology,* **16,** suppl. 32, 54.

—— Tsingoglou, S. (1968) 'The false fontanelle as a practical method of long-term testing of intracranial pressure.' *Developmental Medicine and Child Neurology,* suppl. 16, 17.

—— Hole, R., Wynne, J. M. (1966) 'Treatment of infantile hydrocephalus using the Holter valve: an analysis of 152 consecutive cases.' *Developmental Medicine and Child Neurology,* suppl. 11, 27.

Forrester, R. M. (1968) 'Ethical and social aspects of treatment of spina bifida.' *Lancet,* **ii,** 1033 (Letter).

Foster, F. (1973) *The Geographic Viewpoint in Medical Care Studies.* Ph.D. Thesis. University of Edinburgh.

Fowler, I. (1953) 'Responses of the chick neural tube in mechanically produced spina bifida.' *Journal of Experimental Zoology,* **123,** 115.

Freehafer, A. A., Vessely, J. C., Mack, R. P. (1972) 'Iliopsoas muscle transfer in the treatment of myelomeningocele patients with paralytic hip deformities.' *Journal of Bone and Joint Surgery,* **54A,** 1715.

Freeston, B. M. (1971) 'An enquiry into the effect of a spina bifida child upon family life.' *Developmental Medicine and Child Neurology,* **13,** 456.

Friedman, B., Smith, D. R., Finkle, A. L. (1964) 'Prosthetic bladder of silicone rubber in dogs.' *Investigative Urology,* **1,** 323.

181

Front, D., Overbeek, W. J., Penning, L. (1972) 'The study of infantile hydrocephalus with combined air and isotope ventriculography.' *Journal of Neurology, Neurosurgery and Psychiatry,* **35,** 456.

Garceau, G. J., Brahms, M. A. (1956) 'A preliminary study of selective plantar-muscle denervation of pes cavus.' *Journal of Bone and Joint Surgery,* **38A,** 553.

Gardner, W. J. (1965) 'Hydrodynamic mechanisms of syringomyelia: its relationship to myelocoele.' *Journal of Neurology, Neurosurgery and Psychiatry,* **28,** 247.

—— (1966) 'Embryologic origin of spinal malformations.' *Acta Radiologica,* **5,** 1013.

—— (1968) 'Myelocele: rupture of the neural tube?' *Clinical Neurosurgery,* **15,** 57.

Geoffroy Saint-Hilaire, I. (1836) *Histoire Générale et Particulière des Anomalies de l'Organisation chez l'Homme et les Animaux; Recherches sur les Caractères, les Causes etc. des Monstruosités, des Variétés et des Vices de Conformation ou Traité de Tératologie.* Paris: Baillière.

Giroud, A. (1961) 'Meningocoeles rachidiennes et fermeture imparfaite du tube médullaire.' *Archives d'Anatomie, d'Histologie et d'Embryologie,* **44,** suppl. 1.

—— Martinet, M., Lefebvres-Boisselot, J. (1960) 'Relations entre les anomalies de fermeture du tube nerveux et les déficiences de la voûte osseuse du nevraxe et l'indifférenciation de l'épiderme surjacent.' *Archives d'Anatomie, d'Histologie et d'Embryologie,* **43,** 201.

Goldstein, F., Kepes, J. J. (1966) 'The role of traction in the development of the Arnold-Chiari malformation. An experimental study.' *Journal of Neuropathology and Experimental Neurology,* **25,** 654.

Granholm, L. (1968) 'On water shifts in the hydrocephalic brain.' *Developmental Medicine and Child Neurology,* suppl. 16, 1.

Grice, D. S. (1952) 'An extra-articular arthrodesis of the subastragalar joint for the correction of paralytic flat feet in children.' *Journal of Bone and Joint Surgery,* **34A,** 927.

Grimes, J. H., Anderson, E. E., Currie, D. P. (1973) 'Surgical management of the neurogenic bladder.' *Urology,* **2,** 500.

Gruenwald, P. (1941) 'Tissue anomalies of probable neural crest origin in a 20mm human embryo with myeloschisis.' *Archives of Pathology,* **31,** 489.

Guthkelch, A. N. (1962) 'Studies in spina bifida cystica. III. Seasonal variation in the frequency of spina bifida births.' *British Journal of Preventive and Social Medicine,* **16,** 159.

—— (1964) 'Studies in spina bifida cystica (Part V) Anomalous reflexes in congenital spinal palsy.' *Developmental Medicine and Child Neurology,* **6,** 264.

—— (1974) 'Diastematomyelia with median septum.' *Brain,* **97,** 729.

Guttman, L. (1954) 'Initial treatment of traumatic paraplegia.' *Proceedings of the Royal Society of Medicine,* **47,** 1103.

Hadenius, A. M., Hagberg, B., Hyttnäs-Bensch, K., Sjögren, I. (1962) 'The natural prognosis of infantile hydrocephalus.' *Acta Paediatrica,* **51,** 117.

Hakim, S. (1973) 'Hydraulic and mechanical mis-matching of valve shunts used in the treatment of hydrocephalus: the need for a servo-valve shunt.' *Developmental Medicine and Child Neurology,* **15,** 646.

Halverstadt, D. B., Parry, W. L. (1975) 'Electronic stimulation of the human bladder nine years later.' *Journal of Urology,* **113,** 341.

Hamilton, W. J., Boyd, J. D., Mossman, H. W. (1952) *Human Embryology. (Prenatal development of form and function.) 2nd ed.* Baltimore: Williams and Wilkins.

Hare, E. H., Laurence, K. M., Payne, H., Rawnsley, K. (1966) 'Spina bifida cystica and family stress.' *British Medical Journal,* **ii,** 757.

Hay, M. C., Walker, G. (1973) 'Plantar pressures in healthy children and in children with myelo-meningocele.' *Journal of Bone and Joint Surgery,* **55B,** 828.

Hayden, P. W., Shurtleff, D. B. (1967) 'Reduction of cerebral ventricular hypertension with 1.4:3, dianhydro-D-glucitol.' *Developmental Medicine and Child Neurology,* suppl. 13, 134.

—— —— (1972) 'The medical management of hydrocephalus.' *Developmental Medicine and Child Neurology,* **14,** suppl. 27, 52.

Hayes, J. T., Gross, H. P. (1963) 'Orthopedic implications of myelodysplasia.' *Journal of the American Medical Association,* **184,** 762.

—— —— Dow, S. (1964) 'Surgery for paralytic defects secondary to myelomeningocele and myelodysplasia.' *Journal of Bone and Joint Surgery,* **46A,** 1577.

Hemmer, R. (1967) 'Complications relating to ventriculo-venous shunts: a five year study.' *Developmental Medicine and Child Neurology,* suppl. 13, 108.

Hendren, W. H. (1973) 'Reconstruction of previously diverted urinary tracts in children.' *Journal of Pediatric Surgery,* **8,** 135.

Herzog, E. G., Sharrard, W. J. W. (1966) 'Calipers and brace with double hip locks.' *Clinical Orthopedics,* **46,** 239.

Hewitt, D. (1963) 'Geographical variations in the mortality attributed to spina bifida and other congenital malformations.' *British Journal of Preventive and Social Medicine*, **17**, 13.

Heyman, C. H., Herndon, C. H., Strong, J. M. (1958) 'Mobilization of the tarso-metatarsal and inter-metatarsal joints for the correction of resistant adduction of the fore part of the foot in congenital club-foot or congenital metatarsus varus.' *Journal of Bone and Joint Surgery*, **40A**, 299.

Hide, D. W., Semple, C. (1970) 'Co-ordinated care of the child with spina bifida.' *Lancet*, **ii**, 605.

Hoffer, M. M., Feiwell, E., Perry, R., Perry, J., Bonnett, C. (1973) 'Functional ambulation in patients with myelomeningocele.' *Journal of Bone and Joint Surgery*, **55A**, 137.

Holmdahl, D. E. (1925) 'Die erste Entwicklung des Körpers bei den Vögeln und Säugetieren, inkl. dem Menschen, besonders mit Rücksicht auf die Bildung des Rückenmarks, des Zöloms und der entodermalen Kloake nebst einem Exkurs über die Entstehung der Spina Bifida in der Lumbosakral-region.' *Morphologisches Jahrbuch*, **55**, 112.

Holt, R. J., Newman, R. L. (1972) 'The treatment of urinary candidosis with the oral antifungal drugs 5-fluorocytosine and "Clotrimazole".' *Developmental Medicine and Child Neurology*, suppl. 27, 70.

Holtzer, G. J., de Lange, S. A. (1973) 'Shunt-independent arrest of hydrocephalus.' *Journal of Neurosurgery*, **39**, 698.

Hopkinson, B. R., Hardman, J. (1973) 'Silicone rubber perianal suture for rectal prolapse.' *Proceedings of the Royal Society of Medicine*, **66**, 1095.

—— Lightwood, R. (1967) 'Electrical treatment of incontinence.' *British Journal of Surgery*, **54**, 802.

Hoppenfeld, S. (1967) 'Congenital kyphosis in myelomeningocele.' *Journal of Bone and Joint Surgery*, **49B**, 276.

Howell, D. G. (1967) 'The use of the colonic conduit in the treatment of urinary incontinence in congenital spinal palsy.' *Developmental Medicine and Child Neurology*, suppl. 13, 119.

Humphry, G. M. (1885) 'The anatomy of spina bifida.' *Journal of Anatomy and Physiology*, **19**, 500.

—— (1886) 'Six specimens of spina bifida with bony projections from the bodies of the vertebrae into the vertebral canal.' *Journal of Anatomy and Physiology*, **20**, 585.

Hunt, G., Lewin, W., Gleave, J., Gairdner, D. (1973) 'Predictive factors in open myelomeningocele with special reference to sensory level.' *British Medical Journal*, **iv**, 197.

Hutch, J. A. (1971) 'The internal urinary sphincter: a double-loop system.' *Journal of Urology*, **105**, 375.

Huttenlocher, P. R. (1965) 'Treatment of hydrocephalus with acetazolamide: results in 15 cases.' *Journal of Pediatrics*, **66**, 1023.

Ingraham, F. D., Scott, H. W. (1943) 'Spina bifida and cranium bifidum. The Arnold-Chiari malformation —a study of 20 cases.' *New England Journal of Medicine*, **229**, 108.

Ingram, T. T. S., Naughton, J. A. (1962) 'Paediatric and psychological aspects of cerebral palsy associated with hydrocephalus.' *Developmental Medicine and Child Neurology*, **4**, 287.

James, C. C. M. (1970) 'Fractures of the lower limbs in spina bifida cystica: a survey of 44 fractures in 122 children.' *Developmental Medicine and Child Neurology*, suppl. 22, 88.

—— Lassman, L. P. (1960) 'Spinal dysraphism: an orthopaedic syndrome in children accompanying occult forms.' *Archives of Disease in Childhood*, **35**, 315.

—— —— (1964) 'Diastematomyelia: a critical survey of 24 cases submitted to laminectomy.' *Archives of Disease in Childhood*, **39**, 125.

—— —— (1967) 'Results of treatment of progressive lesions in spina bifida occulta five to ten years after laminectomy.' *Lancet*, **ii**, 1277.

—— —— (1972) *Spinal Dysraphism: Spina Bifida Occulta*. London: Butterworths.

Jelínek, R., Pexieder, T. (1968) 'The pressure of encephalic fluid in chick embryos between the 2nd and 6th day of incubation.' *Physiologia Bohemoslovaca*, **17**, 297.

—— —— (1970) 'Pressure of the CSF and morphogenesis of the CNS. I. Chick embryo.' *Folia Morphologica*, **18**, 102.

Katona, F., Eckstein, H. B. (1974) 'Treatment of neuropathic bladder by transurethral electrical stimulation.' *Lancet*, **i**, 780.

Key, A., Retzius, G. (1875-6) *Studien in der Anatomie des Nervensystems und des Bindgewebes*. Stockholm: Samson and Wallin.

Keys Smith, G., Durham Smith, E. (1973) 'Selection for treatment in spina bifida cystica.' *British Medical Journal*, **iv**, 189.

Kimmel, G. C. (1942) 'Hypertension and pyelonephritis of children.' *American Journal of the Diseases of Children*, **63**, 60.

Kirkland, I. (1962) 'Urinary tract problems in spina bifida.' *Developmental Medicine and Child Neurology*, **4**, 314.

Kruyff, E., Jeffs, R. (1966) 'Skull abnormalities associated with the Arnold-Chiari malformation.' *Acta Radiologica*, **5**, 9.

Laurence, K. M. (1964) 'The natural history of spina bifida cystica. Detailed analysis of 407 cases.' *Archives of Disease in Childhood*, **39**, 41.

—— (1966) 'The survival of untreated spina bifida cystica.' *Developmental Medicine and Child Neurology*, suppl. 1, 10.

—— (1969) 'The recurrence risk in spina bifida cystica and anencephaly.' *Developmental Medicine and Child Neurology*, suppl. 20, 23.

—— Carter, C. O., David, P. A. (1968a) 'Major central nervous system malformations in South Wales. I. Incidence, local variations and geographical factors.' *British Journal of Preventive and Social Medicine*, **22**, 146.

—— —— —— (1968b) 'Major central nervous system malformations in South Wales. II. Pregnancy factors, seasonal variation, and social class effects.' *British Journal of Preventive and Social Medicine*, **22**, 212.

—— Tew, B. J. (1966) 'Follow-up of 65 survivors from the 425 cases of spina bifida born in South Wales between 1956 and 1962.' *Developmental Medicine and Child Neurology*, suppl. 13, 1.

Lebedeff, A. (1881) 'Ueber die Entstehung der Anencephalie und Spina bifida bei Vögeln und Menschen.' *Virchow's Archiv für pathologische Anatomie und Physiologie und für klinische Medizin*, **86**, 263.

—— (1882) *Lehrbuch des allgemeinen pathologische Anatomie.* p. 297.

Lemire, R. J., Shepard, T. H., Alvord, E. C. (1965) 'Caudal myeloschisis (lumbo-sacral spina bifida cystica) in a five millimeter (Horizon XIV) human embryo.' *Anatomical Record*, **152**, 9.

Lendon, R. G. (1968a) 'Studies on the embryogenesis of spina bifida in the rat.' *Developmental Medicine and Child Neurology*, suppl. 16, 54.

—— (1968b) 'Neuron population in the spinal cord of children with spina bifida and hydrocephalus.' *Developmental Medicine and Child Neurology*, suppl. 15, 50.

—— (1969) 'Neuron population in the lumbosacral cord of myelomeningocele children.' *Developmental Medicine and Child Neurology*, suppl. 20, 82.

—— Ráliš, Z. (1971) 'Normal posture and deformities of the lower limbs in rat fetuses with experimentally produced spina bifida.' *Developmental Medicine and Child Neurology*, suppl. 25, 50.

—— Zachary, R. B. (1974) 'A histological study of the external sphincter in the male infant.' *Developmental Medicine and Child Neurology*, **16**, suppl. 32, 79.

Lichtenstein, B. W. (1940) '"Spinal dysraphism"; spina bifida and myelodysplasia.' *Archives of Neurology and Psychiatry*, **44**, 792.

—— (1942) 'Distant neuroanatomic complications of spina bifida (spinal dysraphism). Hydrocephalus, Arnold-Chiari deformity, stenosis of the aqueduct of Sylvius, etc. Pathogenesis and pathology.' *Archives of Neurology and Psychiatry*, **47**, 195.

Lightowler, C. D. R. (1971) 'Meningomyelocele: the price of treatment.' *British Medical Journal*, **ii**, 385.

Linder, R. (1970) 'Mothers of disabled children—the value of weekly group meetings.' *Developmental Medicine and Child Neurology*, **12**, 202.

Lister, J. (1969) 'The urinary tract in myelomeningocele.' *In* Wilkinson, A. W. (Ed.) *Recent Advances in Paediatric Surgery, 2nd ed.* London: Churchill.

Lorber, J. (1961) 'Systematic ventriculographic studies in infants born with meningomyelocele and encephalocele. The incidence and development of hydrocephalus.' *Archives of Disease in Childhood*, **36**, 381.

—— (1965) 'The family of spina bifida cystica.' *Pediatrics*, **35**, 589.

—— (1971) 'Results of treatment of myelomeningocele. An analysis of 524 unselected cases with special reference to possible selection for treatment.' *Developmental Medicine and Child Neurology*, **13**, 279.

—— (1972) 'The use of isosorbide in the treatment of hydrocephalus.' *Developmental Medicine and Child Neurology*, suppl. 27, 87.

—— (1973a) 'Early results of selective treatment of spina bifida cystica.' *British Medical Journal*, **iv**, 201.

—— (1973b) 'Isosorbide in the medical treatment of infantile hydrocephalus.' *Journal of Neurosurgery*, **39**, 702.

—— Formby, D. (1968) 'Treatment of persistent urinary tract infections with gentamicin.' *Developmental Medicine and Child Neurology*, suppl. 16, 93.

—— Menneer, P. C., Allott, D. C. (1968) 'An investigation into prophylactic treatment of urinary tract infections in infants born with spina bifida cystica.' *Developmental Medicine and Child Neurology*, suppl. 15, 30.

—— Schloss, A. L. (1973) 'The adolescent with myelomeningocele.' *Developmental Medicine and Child Neurology*, suppl. 29, 113.

Luschka, H. von (1854) 'Zur Lehre von der Sekretionstelle.' *Archiv für physiologische Heilkunde*, **13**, 1.

—— (1855) *Die Adergeflechte des menschlichen Gehirnes.* Berlin: G. Reimer.

Luthardt, T. (1970) 'Bacterial infections in ventriculo-auricular shunt systems.' *Developmental Medicine and Child Neurology,* **12,** suppl.22, 105.

McCoy, W. T., Simpson, D. A., Carter, R. F. (1967) 'Cerebral malformations complicating spina bifida. Radiological studies.' *Clinical Radiology,* **18,** 176.

McHaffie, G. (1974) Personal communication to Dr. Gordon Stark.

Mac Keith, R. (1973) 'The feelings and behaviour of parents of handicapped children.' *Developmental Medicine and Child Neurology,* **15,** 524.

Mackenzie, N. G., Emery, J. L. (1971) 'Deformities of the cervical cord in children with neurospinal dysraphism.' *Developmental Medicine and Child Neurology,* suppl. 25, 58.

McKeown, T., Record, R. G. (1960) 'Malformations in a population observed 5 years after birth.' *In* Wolstenholme, G. E. W., O'Connor, C. M. (Eds.) *Ciba Foundation Symposium on Congenital Malformations.* London: Churchill, p. 2.

McKibbin, B. (1973) 'The use of splintage in the management of paralytic dislocation of the hip in spina bifida cystica.' *Journal of Bone and Joint Surgery,* **55B,** 163.

McKibbin, B., Porter, R. W. (1967) 'The incidence of vitamin-C deficiency in meningomyelocele.' *Developmental Medicine and Child Neurology,* **9,** 338.

—— Toseland, T. A., Duckworth, T. (1968) 'Abnormalities in vitamin C metabolism in spina bifida.' *Developmental Medicine and Child Neurology,* suppl. 15, 55.

Magendie, F. (1825) 'Mémoire sur le liquide qui se trouve dans le crâne et l'épine de l'homme et des animaux vertébrés.' *Journal de Physiologie Expérimentale,* **5,** 27.

—— (1827) 'Mémoire sur le liquide qui se trouve dans le crâne et l'épine de l'homme et des animaux vertébrés.' *Journal de Physiologie Expérimentale,* **7,** 1, 17, 66.

—— (1828) 'Mémoire physiologique sur le cerveau.' *Journal de Physiologie Expérimentale,* **8,** 211.

—— (1842) 'Recherches physiologiques et cliniques sur le liquide céphalo-rachidien ou cérébrospinal.' Paris: J. B. Bailliere.

Malament, M. (1972) 'External sphincterotomy in neurogenic bladder dysfunction.' *Journal of Urology,* **108,** 554.

Marsh, H., Gould, A. P., Clutton, H. H., Parker, R. W. (1885) 'Report of a Committee of the Society nominated Nov.10 1882 to investigate spina bifida and its treatment by the injection of Dr. Morton's iodoglycerine solution.' *Transactions of the Clinical Society of London,* **18,** 339.

Martin, M. C. (1964) 'Physiotherapy in relation to myelomeningocele.' *Physiotherapy,* **50,** 50.

—— (1967) 'Spina bifida.' *Physiotherapy,* **53,** 299.

Mawdsley, T., Rickham, P. O., Roberts, J. R. (1967) 'Long-term results of early operation of open myelomeningoceles and encephaloceles.' *British Medical Journal,* **i,** 663.

Mayo-Robson, A. W. (1885) 'A series of cases of spina bifida treated by plastic operation.' *Transactions of the Clinical Society of London,* **18,** 210.

Mealey, J., Barker, D. T. (1968) 'Failure of oral acetazolamide to avert hydrocephalus in infants with myelomeningocele.' *Journal of Pediatrics,* **72,** 257.

Menelaus, M. B. (1971*a*) *The Orthopaedic Management of Spina Bifida Cystica.* Edinburgh: Livingstone.

—— (1971*b*) 'Talectomy for equinovarus deformity in arthrogryposis and spina bifida.' *Journal of Bone and Joint Surgery,* **53B,** 468.

Merrill, D. C., Conway, C. J. (1974) 'Clinical experience with the Mentor bladder stimulator: I. Patients with upper motor neuron lesions.' *Journal of Urology,* **112,** 52.

Millin, T., Read, C. D. (1948) 'Stress incontinence of urine in the female: Part II. Millin's sling operation.' *Postgraduate Medical Journal,* **24,** 51.

Miller, E., Sethi, L. (1971) 'The effect of hydrocephalus on perception.' *Developmental Medicine and Child Neurology,* suppl. 25, 77.

Milhorat, T. H. (1972) *Hydrocephalus and the Cerebrospinal Fluid.* Baltimore: Williams and Wilkins.

—— Mosher, M. B. (1970) 'Choroid plexectomy: a clinical and experimental study.' Paper delivered at meeting of Cushing Society (The American Association of Neurological Surgeons). April 1970.

—— Hammock, M. K., Di Chiro, G. (1971) 'The subarachnoid space in congenital obstructive hydrocephalus. Part I. Cisternographic findings.' *Journal of Neurosurgery,* **35,** 1.

Mogg, R. A. (1967) 'Treatment of urinary incontinence using the colonic conduit.' *Journal of Urology,* **97,** 684.

Morgagni, J. B. (1761) *The seats and causes of diseases investigated by anatomy.* Trans. by William Cooke 1822. London: Longman, p. 23.

Morton, J. (1877) *Treatment of Spina Bifida by a New Method.* Glasgow: J. Maclehose.

—— (1887) *Treatment of Spina Bifida by a New Method. With a Paper on the Pathology of Spina Bifida,* by John Clelland. London: Churchill.

Naggan, L. (1971) 'Anencephaly and spina bifida in Israel.' *Pediatrics,* **47,** 577.

—— MacMahon, B. (1971) 'Ethnic differences in the prevalence of anencephaly and spina bifida in Boston, Massachusetts.' *New England Journal of Medicine,* **277,** 1119.

Naik, D. R., Emery, J. L. (1968) 'The position of the spinal cord segments related to the vertebral bodies in children with meningomyelocele and hydrocephalus.' *Developmental Medicine and Child Neurology,* suppl. 16, 62.

Nanninga, J. B., Rosen, J., O'Conor, V. J. (1974) 'Experience with transurethral external sphincterotomy in patients with spinal cord injury.' *Journal of Urology,* **112,** 72.

Nash, D. F. E. (1956) 'Ileal loop bladder in congenital spinal palsy.' *British Journal of Urology,* **28,** 387.

—— (1970) 'The impact of the total care with special reference to myelodysplasia.' *Developmental Medicine and Child Neurology,* suppl. 22, 1.

Nashold, B. S., Friedman, H., Boyarsky, S. (1971) 'Electrical activation of micturition by spinal cord stimulation.' *Journal of Surgical Research,* **11,** 144.

Neel, J. V. (1958) 'A study of major congenital defects in Japanese infants.' *American Journal of Human Genetics,* **10,** 398.

Nellhaus, G. (1968) 'Head circumference from birth to eighteen years.' *Paediatrics,* **41,** 114.

Nelson, J. D., Peters, P. C. (1965) 'Supra-pubic aspiration of urine in premature and term infants.' *Pediatrics,* **36,** 132.

Nergårdh, A., Hedenberg, C. von, Hellström, B., Ericsson, N.-O. (1974) 'Continence training of children with neurogenic bladder dysfunction.' *Developmental Medicine and Child Neurology,* **16,** 47.

Nicholas, J. L., Kamal, I. M., Eckstein, H. B. (1970) 'Immediate shunt replacement in the treatment of bacterial colonisation of Holter valves.' *Developmental Medicine and Child Neurology,* suppl. 22, 110.

Nicholas, J. L. (1972) Unpublished data.

Nixon, H. H. (1969) 'Devices for bladder and bowel control.' *In* Wilkinson, A. W. (Ed.) *Recent Advances in Pediatric Surgery, 2nd ed.* London: Churchill.

—— (1975) Personal communication.

—— Kapila, L. (1968) 'A technique for urinary diversion.' *Developmental Medicine and Child Neurology,* suppl. 16, 108.

Norrell, H., Wilson, C., Howieson, J., Megison, L., Bertan, V. (1969) 'Venous factors in infantile hydrocephalus.' *Journal of Neurosurgery,* **31,** 561.

Ogryzlo, M. A. (1942) 'The Arnold-Chiari malformation.' *Archives of Neurology and Psychiatry,* **48,** 30.

Ostertag, B. (1956) *Handbuch der speziellen pathologischen natomie und Histologie,* Vol. XII, p. 285.

Padget, D. H. (1968) 'Spina bifida and embryonic neuroschisis—a causal relationship. Definition of the postnatal conformations involving a bifid spine.' *Johns Hopkins Medical Journal,* **123,** 233.

—— (1970) 'Neuroschisis and human embryonic maldevelopment. New evidence on anencephaly, spina bifida and diverse mammalian defects.' *Journal of Neuropathology and Experimental Neurology,* **29,** 192.

Paquin, A. J. (1959) 'Ureterovesical anastomosis: the description and evaluation of a technique.' *Journal of Urology,* 82, 573.

Parsons, J. G. (1968) 'An investigation into the verbal facility of hydrocephalic children, with special reference to vocabulary, morphology and fluency.' *Developmental Medicine and Child Neurology,* suppl. 16, 109.

—— (1969) 'Short-term verbal memory in hydrocephalic children.' *Developmental Medicine and Child Neurology,* suppl. 20, 75.

—— (1972) 'Assessments of aptitudes in young people of school-leaving age handicapped by hydrocephalus or spina bifida cystica.' *Developmental Medicine and Child Neurology,* suppl. 27, 101.

Patten, B. M. (1953) 'Embryological states in the establishing of myeloschisis with spina bifida.' *American Journal of Anatomy,* **93,** 365.

Paul, S. W. (1972) 'Bracing in myelomeningocele.' *In American Academy of Orthopaedic Surgeons, a Symposium on Myelomeningocele.* St. Louis: C. V. Mosby, p. 219.

Pekarovič, E., Robinson, A., Lister, J., Zachary, R. B. (1968) 'Pressure variations in intestinal loops used for urinary diversion.' *Developmental Medicine and Child Neurology,* suppl. 16, 87.

—— Zachary, R. B., Lister, J. (1970) 'Indications for manual expression of the neurogenic bladder.' *British Journal of Urology,* **42,** 191.

Penfield, W., Coburn, D. F. (1938) 'Arnold-Chiari malformation and its operative treatment.' *Archives of Neurology and Psychiatry,* **40,** 328.

Pickrell, K., Georgiade, N., Crawford, H., Maguire, C., Boone, A. (1956) 'Gracilis muscle transplant for correction of urinary incontinence in male children.' *Annals of Surgery,* **143,** 764.

Politano, V. A., Leadbetter, W. F. (1958) 'An operative technique for the correction of vesicoureteral reflux.' *Journal of Urology,* **79,** 573.

Porter, R. W. (1968) 'Vasomotor control in the lower limbs of children with meningomyeloceles.' *Developmental Medicine and Child Neurology,* suppl. 15, 62.

186

Pryles, C. V., Atkin, M. D., Morse, T. S., Welch, K. J. (1959) 'Comparative bacteriologic study of urine obtained from children by percutaneous suprapubic aspiration of the bladder and by catheter.' *Pediatrics*, **24**, 983.

Ráliš, Z. (1970) 'Muscle morphology in spina bifida hip deformities'. *Developmental Medicine and Child Neurology*, suppl. 22, 137.

—— (1974) 'Intra-uterine development of lower limb deformities in spina bifida.' Paper presented to the meeting of the Society for Research into Spina Bifida and Hydrocephalus. Gothenburg, 1974.

Record, R. G., McKeown, T. (1949) 'Congenital malformation of the central nervous system. I. A survey of 930 cases.' *British Journal of Preventive and Social Medicine*, **3**, 183.

Renwick, J. H. (1972) 'Hypothesis: anencephaly and spina bifida are usually preventable by avoidance of a specific but unidentified substance present in certain potato tubers.' *British Journal of Preventive and Social Medicine*, **26**, 67.

Richards, I. D. G., Roberts, C. J., Lloyd, S. (1972) 'Area differences in prevalence of neural tube malformations in South Wales. A study of possible demographic determinants.' *British Journal of Preventive and Social Medicine*, **26**, 89.

—— McIntosh, H. T. (1973) 'Spina bifida survivors and their parents: a study of problems and services.' *Developmental Medicine and Child Neurology*, **15**, 293.

Rickham, P. P. (1964) 'Permanent urinary diversion in childhood.' *Annals of the Royal College of Surgeons*, **35**, 84.

—— Mawdsley, T. (1966) 'The effect of early operation on the survival of spina bifida cystica.' *Developmental Medicine and Child Neurology*, suppl. 11, 20.

Roberts, J. B. M. (1962) 'Spina bifida and the urinary tract.' *Annals of the Royal College of Surgeons*, **31**, 69.

Recklinghausen, F. von (1886) 'Untersuchungen über die Spina bifida.' *Virchows Archiv für pathologische Anatomie und Physiologie und für klinische Medizin*, **105**, 243.

Ruben, R. C., Henderson, E. S., Ommaya, A. K., Walker, M. D., Rall, D. P. (1966) 'The production of cerebrospinal fluid in man and its modification by acetazolamide.' *Journal of Neurosurgery*, **25**, 430.

Rueda, J., Carroll, N. C. (1972) 'Hip instability in patients with myelomeningocele.' *Journal of Bone and Joint Surgery*, **54B**, 422.

Russell, D. S., Donald, C. (1935) 'The mechanism of internal hydrocephalus in spina bifida.' *Brain*, **58**, 203.

Scarff, J. E. (1963) 'Treatment of hydrocephalus: an historical and critical review of methods and results.' *Journal of Neurology, Neurosurgery and Psychiatry*, **26**, 1.

Schaltenbrand, G. (1955) 'Plexus und Meningen.' *In* Moellendorff, W. von (Ed.) *Handbuch der Mikroskopischen Anatomie des Menschen. Nervensystem*, vol.IV/2. Berlin: Springer.

Schwalbe, E., Gredig, M. (1907) 'Über Entwicklungsstörungen des Kleinhirns, Hirnstamms und Halsmarks bei Spina bifida. (Arnold'sche und Chiari'sche Missbildung.)' *Beitraege zur pathologischen Anatomie*, **40**, 132.

Scott, F. B., Bradley, W. E., Timm, G. W. (1974) 'Treatment of urinary incontinence by an implantable prosthetic urinary sphincter.' *Journal of Urology*, **112**, 75.

Sharrard, W. J. W. (1962) 'The mechanism of paralytic deformity in spina bifida.' *Developmental Medicine and Child Neurology*, **4**, 310.

—— (1964a) 'The segmental innervation of the lower limb muscles in man.' *Annals of the Royal College of Surgeons*, **35**, 106.

—— (1964b) 'Posterior iliopsoas transplantation in the treatment of paralytic dislocation of the hip.' *Journal of Bone and Joint Surgery*, **46B**, 426.

—— (1967) 'Paralytic deformity in the lower limb.' *Journal of Bone and Joint Surgery*, **49B**, 731.

—— (1968) 'Spinal osteotomy for congenital kyphosis in myelomingocele.' *Journal of Bone and Joint Surgery*, **50B**, 466.

—— (1971) *Paediatric Orthopaedics and Fractures*. Oxford: Blackwell Scientific Publications.

—— (1973) 'The orthopaedic surgery of spina bifida.' *Clinical Orthopedics*, **92**, 195.

—— Drennan, J. C. (1972) 'Osteotomy-excision of the spine for lumbar kyphosis in older children with myelomeningocele.' *Journal of Bone and Joint Surgery*, **54B**, 50.

—— Webb, J. (1974) 'Supra-malleolar wedge osteotomy of the tibia in children with myelomeningocele.' *Journal of Bone and Joint Surgery*, **56B**, 458.

—— Zachary, R. B., Lorber, J. (1967) 'Survival and paralysis in open myelomeningocele with special reference to the time of repair of the spinal lesion.' *Developmental Medicine and Child Neurology*, suppl. 13, 35.

—— —— —— Bruce, A. M. (1963) 'A controlled trial of immediate and delayed closure of spina bifida cystica.' *Archives of Disease in Childhood*, **38**, 18.

187

Smith, C. (1972) 'Computer programmes to estimate recurrence risks for multi-factorial familial disease.' *British Medical Journal*, **i,** 495.

Smith, E. D. (1965) *Spina Bifida and the Total Care of Spina Myelomeningocele.* Springfield, Ill.: C. C. Thomas.

—— (1972*a*) 'Urinary prognosis in spina bifida.' *Journal of Urology*, **108,** 815.

—— (1972*b*) 'Follow-up studies on 150 ileal conduits in children.' *Journal of Pediatric Surgery*, **7,** 1.

Smith, T. W. D., Sharrard, W. J. W. (1973) 'Flexor hallucis longus tenodesis: a new operation for clawing of the hallux.' *Journal of Bone and Joint Surgery*, **55B,** 879.

Smithells, R. W. (1967) Personal communication quoted by Laurence (1969).

—— D'Arcy, E. E., McAllister, E. F. (1968) 'The outcome of pregnancies before and after the birth of infants with nervous system malformations.' *Developmental Medicine and Child Neurology*, suppl. 15, 6.

Snow, J. B., Rogers, K. A. (1965) 'Bilateral abductor paralysis of the vocal chords secondary to the Arnold-Chiari malformation and its management.' *Laryngoscope*, **75,** 316.

Sriram, K., Bobechko, W. P., Hall, J. E. (1972) 'Surgical management of spinal deformities in spina bifida.' *Journal of Bone and Joint Surgery*, **54B,** 666.

Stark, G. D. (1968*a*) 'Pathophysiology of the bladder in myelomeningocele and its correlation with the neurological picture.' *Developmental Medicine and Child Neurology*, suppl. 16, 76.

—— (1968*b*) 'Treatment of ventriculitis in hydrocephalic infants: intrathecal and intraventricular use of the new penicillins.' *Developmental Medicine and Child Neurology*, suppl. 15, 36.

—— (1971) 'Neonatal assessment of the child with myelomeningocele.' *Archives of Disease in Childhood*, **46,** 539.

—— (1973) 'Correlative studies of bladder function in myelomeningocele.' *Developmental Medicine and Child Neurology*, suppl. 29, 55.

—— Baker, G. C. W. (1967) 'The neurological involvement of the lower limbs in myelomeningocele.' *Developmental Medicine and Child Neurology*, **9,** 732.

—— Drummond, M. (1971) 'The spinal cord lesion in myelomeningocele.' *Developmental Medicine and Child Neurology*, suppl. 25, 1.

—— —— (1972) 'Results of selective early operation for myelomeningocele.' *Developmental Medicine and Child Neurology*, suppl. 27, 155.

—— —— (1973) 'Results of selective early operation in myelomeningocele.' *Archives of Disease in Childhood*, **48,** 676.

Sternberg, H. (1929) 'Über Spaltbildungen des Medullarrohres bei jungen menschlichen Embryonen, ein Beitrag zur Entstehung der Anencephalie und der Rachischisis.' *Virchows Archiv für pathologische Anatomie und Physiologie und für klinische Medizin*, **272,** 325.

Stevenson, A. C., Johnston, H. A., Stewart, M. I. P., Golding, D. R. (1966) 'Congenital malformations. A report of a study of a series of consecutive births in 24 centres.' *Bulletin of the World Health Organization*, **34,** suppl. 9, 127.

—— Warnock, H. A. (1959) 'Observations on the results of pregnancies of women in Belfast. 1. Data relating to all pregnancies ending in 1957.' *Annals of Human Genetics*, **23,** 382.

Strach, E. H. (1972) 'The spring implant operation: a preliminary report.' *Developmental Medicine and Child Neurology*, suppl. 27, 121.

Swinyard, C. A., Shahani, B. T. (1966) *In Comprehensive Care of the Child with Spina Bifida Manifesta. Rehabilitation Monograph XXXI.* New York: New York University Bellvue Medical Center.

Taylor, R. G. (1951) 'The treatment of claw toes by multiple transfers of flexor into extensor tendons.' *Journal of Bone and Joint Surgery*, **33B,** 539.

Tew, B., Laurence, K. M. (1973) 'Mothers, brothers and sisters of patients with spina bifida.' *Developmental Medicine and Child Neurology*, suppl. 29, 69.

Tew, B. J., Payne, H., Laurence, K. M. (1974) 'Must a family with a handicapped child be a handicapped family?' *Developmental Medicine and Child Neurology*, suppl. 32, 95.

Thomas, G., Shapiro, S. R., Johnston, J. H. (1975) 'Ureteral reimplantation in children with neurogenic vesical dysfunction.' (In press.)

—— Zachary, R. B., Lister, J. (1974) '"Closed" external sphincterotomy for bladder outlet obstruction in myelomeningocele.' *British Journal of Urology*, **45,** 515.

Timm, G. W., Bradley, W. E. (1971) 'Electromechanical restoration of the micturition reflex.' *IEEE Transactions of Biomedical Engineering*, **18,** 274.

Tribe, C. R. (1963) 'Causes of death in the early and late stages of paraplegia.' *Paraplegia*, **1,** 19.

Tsingoglou, S., Forrest, D. M. (1968) 'Therapeutic and prophylactic lengthening of distal catheter of the Holter ventriculo-atrial shunt.' *Developmental Medicine and Child Neurology*, suppl. 16, 35.

Tulp, N. (1652) *Observationes Medicae.* Amsterdam.

Tzimas, N. A. (1966) 'Orthopaedic care of the child with spina bifida.' *In Comprehensive Care of the Child with Spina Bifida Manifesta. Rehabilitation Monograph XXXI.* New York: New York University, Bellvue Medical Center.

Van Houweninge Graftdijk (1932) Thesis. Leyden University. Personal communication and translation from Dr. K. G. Go of Groningen.

Van Hoytema, G. J., van den Berg, R. (1966) 'Embryological studies of the posterior fossa in connection with Arnold-Chiari malformation.' *Developmental Medicine and Child Neurology,* suppl. 11, 61.

Variend, S., Emery, J. L. (1973) 'The weight of the cerebellum in children with myelomeningocele.' *Developmental Medicine and Child Neurology,* suppl. 29, 77.

—— —— (1974) 'Deformities of the central lobes of the cerebellum in children with myelomeningoceles.' *Developmental Medicine and Child Neurology,* suppl. 32, 99.

Verrier Jones, E. R., Williams, J. E. (1966) 'Urinary investigations in spina bifida cystica during the first month of life.' *Developmental Medicine and Child Neurology,* suppl. 13, 113.

Vincent, S. A. (1966) 'Some aspects of bladder mechanics.' *Biomedical Engineering,* **1**, 438.

Virchow, R. (1863) 'Die Betheiligung des Rückenmarkes an der Spina bifida und die hydromyelie.' *Archiv für pathologische Anatomie und Physiologie,* **27**, 575.

Vogt, E. C., Wyatt, G. M. (1941) 'Craniolacunia (lückenschadel): report of 54 cases.' *Radiology,* **36**, 147.

Wald, N. S., Brock, D. J. H., Bonnar, J. (1974) 'Prenatal diagnosis of spina bifida and anencephaly by maternal serum alphafeto-protein measurement. A controlled study.' *Lancet,* **i**, 765.

Walker, G. (1971) 'The early management of varus feet in myelomeningocele.' *Journal of Bone and Joint Surgery,* **53B**, 462.

—— Cheong-Leem, P. (1973) 'The surgical management of paralytic vertical talus in myelomeningocele.' *Developmental Medicine and Child Neurology,* suppl. 29, 112.

Walker, J. H., Thomas, M., Russell, I. T. (1971) 'Spina bifida—and the parents.' *Developmental Medicine and Child Neurology,* **13**, 462.

Wallace, S. J. (1973) 'The effect of the upper-limb function on mobility of children with myelomeningocele.' *Developmental Medicine and Child Neurology,* suppl. 29, 84.

Warkany, J. (1971) *Congenital Malformations, Notes and Comments.* Chicago: Yearbook Medical Publishers.

—— Wilson, J. G., Geiger, J. F. (1958) 'Myeloschisis and myelomeningocele produced experimentally in the rat.' *Journal of Comparative Neurology,* **109**, 35.

Waterston, J. (1923) 'Annotation.' *Proceedings of the Anatomical Society of Great Britain and Ireland,* **57**, 67.

Wealthall, S. R., Whittaker, G. E., Greenwood, N. (1974) 'The relationship of apnoea and stridor in spina bifida to other unexplained infant deaths.' *Developmental Medicine and Child Neurology,* suppl. 32. 107.

Weed, L. H. (1917) 'The development of the cerebrospinal spaces in pig and in man.' *Contributions to Embryology,* **5**, 3.

—— (1922) 'The absorption of cerebrospinal fluid into the venous system.' *American Journal of Anatomy,* **31**, 191.

—— (1938) 'Meninges and cerebrospinal fluid.' *Journal of Anatomy,* **72**, 181.

Weisl, H., Matthews, J. P. (1973) 'Posterior ilio-psoas transfer in the management of the hip in spina bifida: a review of thirty-four operations.' *Developmental Medicine and Child Neurology,* suppl. 29, 100.

Weller, R. O., Wisniewski, H., Ishii, M., Shulman, D., Terry, R. D. (1969) 'Brain tissue damage in hydrocephalus.' *Developmental Medicine and Child Neurology,* suppl. 20, 1.

Wilcock, A. R., Emery, J. L. (1970) 'Deformities of the renal tract in children with meningomyelocele and hydrocephalus, compared with those of children showing no such central nervous system deformities.' *British Journal of Urology,* **42**, 152.

Williams, B. (1973) 'Is aqueduct stenosis a result of hydrocephalus?' *Brain,* **96**, 399.

Williamson, E. M. (1965) 'Incidence and family aggregation of major congenital malformations of central nervous system.' *Journal of Medical Genetics,* **2**, 161.

Wilson, D. S. (1968) 'Value of preoperative electrodiagnosis in assessment of locomotor function of lower limbs in spina bifida cystica.' *Developmental Medicine and Child Neurology,* suppl. 16, 111.

Wilson, J. T. (1936) 'On the nature and mode of formation of the Foramen of Magendie.' *Journal of Anatomy,* **71**, 423.

Woodburn, M. F. (1974) *Social Implications of Spina Bifida—a Study in South-East Scotland.* Edinburgh: Scottish Spina Bifida Association.

Zachary, R. B. (1966) 'An appraisal of the surgery for meningocele.' *Clinical Neurosurgery,* **13**, 313.

189

Subject Index

U

ulceration 7, 112, 116, 117
upper limbs 163
ureteric implant 140
ureterostomy 140
urethral pressure profile 134
urinary antiseptics 131
urinary obstruction 127
urinary tract infection 22, 64, 126, 143
urinary tract malformations 11, 33, 125
urine testing 132

V

valvular action 18
vaso-motor function 91
vein of Galen 25, 33
veins
  cerebral 33, 45

emissary 33, 45
  frontal 45
  parietal 45
ventral spina bifida 23, 25, 34
ventricular diverticula 39
ventriculo-atrial shunt 38, 39, 45, 72, 73, 77
ventriculo-peritoneal shunt 38, 39, 73, 76, 77
ventriculostomy 37
verbosity 45
vertical talus deformity 88
visuo-spatial relationships 46
vocal cords 44, 45

W

walking training 97, 119 et seq.
welfare 161
wheelchair 92, 112, 121
wound infection 63